TIPS TO KEEP

- What, where, w[...]
  all the difference in the way you feel and look. Improving eating habits may actually make giving up
  cigarettes easier. The four-week diet plan, with
  menus and recipes, shows you how.
- Never smoke while walking. Later on, walking will
  be one of the ways you resist the urge to smoke, so
  start now to associate walking with *not smoking*.

QUITTING

- Combat the oral dilemma by brushing your teeth. It
  not only helps to end a meal, but also gives your
  mouth the impression it has had something sweet to
  eat.
- Drink a cup of warm milk before bedtime to banish
  insomnia. A substance called tryptophan, which occurs naturally in milk, will calm your nerves.

MAINTENANCE

- In the face of an unexpected craving, say: "I've decided not to smoke today," rather than, "I'm never
  going to smoke another cigarette as long as I live."
- Reward yourself. Make sure to spend the money you
  save on cigarettes on special, personal treats.

MARGUERITE THOMAS is a regular contributor to *Prevention* magazine and the author of a cookbook, *The Elegant Peasant*. CAROLINE ADLER has written for *Queen-Harper's* and *London Life*, and is now a freelance writer and video director in New York. Consultant Joël Grinker, Ph.D., is Chairman of the Human Nutrition Department, University of Michigan.

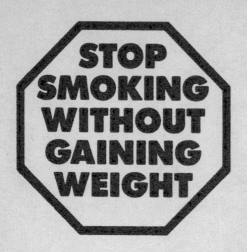

STOP SMOKING WITHOUT GAINING WEIGHT

Caroline Adler
and
Marguerite Thomas

POCKET BOOKS

New York   London   Toronto   Sydney   Tokyo

An *Original* Publication of POCKET BOOKS

POCKET BOOKS, a division of Simon & Schuster Inc.
1230 Avenue of the Americas, New York, NY 10020

ISBN: 0-671-66083-7

First Pocket Books printing January 1989

10 9 8 7 6 5 4 3 2 1

POCKET and colophon are trademarks of
Simon & Schuster Inc.

Printed in the U.S.A.

Contents

Contents

Contents

Preface

Since many individuals who give up smoking do gain weight, it is important to outline a strategy ahead of time to avoid weight gain as well as one for giving up cigarettes. This book presents a safe and effective strategy for dealing with both the problem of smoking cessation and that of potential weight gain.

The Surgeon General of the United States has finally publicly recognized that smoking is an addictive disorder. The addiction, of course, is related to the nicotine content of cigarettes. Recent data suggest that adult smoking has decreased but that significant numbers of young people—especially young women—are starting to smoke. Cigarette advertising, with its picture of sophistication and slimness, may be one of the major reasons why young women take up smoking. But like the majority of the more mature men and women who smoke, they, too, will find it difficult to stop.

Stopping smoking is critical to reduce the health risks of cardiovascular disease, hypertension, and lung cancer. Yet many individuals fail to stop because of a fear of weight gain. Cessation of smoking can be life-saving, but it is also demanding and painful. *Stop Smoking Without Gaining Weight*, outlines a well-thought-out approach to smoking cessation and addresses a major fear—especially among women—that weight gain is inevitable.

Cigarette smoking is correlated with lower body weight and facilitates caloric expenditure. These effects have variously been attributed to reduced caloric intake, increased caloric expenditure, increased metabolic rate, higher sympathetic nervous system activity, and decreased efficiency in caloric storage. A review of the metabolic consequences of smoking will help you to understand the lower body weight of smokers and the frequent weight gain following smoking cessation.

Studies have demonstrated that smoking cessation produces a real and measurable decrease in metabolic rate, increased caloric efficiency or storage of fat, and increased appetite. However, these studies are not conclusive; larger numbers of individuals need to be examined over longer time periods.

While it is clear that increased caloric intake can lead to weight gain, decreased metabolic rates or increased efficiency in caloric storage may be the most significant factors in weight gain. Thus, the postsmoker is not unlike the previously obese individual in that both often have reductions in metabolic rates and feel calorically restricted.

Clearly, information and preparation are essential if the smoker is to quit successfully. This book provides helpful information on smoking cessation techniques and attitude changes. It addresses dietary concerns and proposes an eating program that can be included as part of the strategy to be used against weight gain brought on by smoking cessation. The diet may be safely followed, as it does not recommend severe caloric restriction. By recommending a full range of foods, this program does not risk nutritional deficiencies. Most important, this book recommends exercise rather than low-calorie dieting as a means of preventing weight gain. Most experts in the area of weight control today agree that exercise is the safest and most effective way of preventing weight gain.

By helping the reader address concerns about weight gain in advance, this book can help prevent the crash dieting that often occurs when individuals discover they have gained weight after quitting smoking. The information about attitude change, food concerns, and exercise included in the book will inform and prepare the serious reader. Armed with the knowledge of the physical and psychological effects of quitting smoking, and the benefits of exercise and proper nutrition, the smoker can successfully become the non-smoker.

Dr. Joël A. Grinker
Professor and Director
Program in Human Nutrition
School of Public Health
University of Michigan
Ann Arbor, MI

Foreword

Confessions
of an Ex-Smoker

I don't think of myself as a particularly self-destructive person. You probably don't think of yourself that way either. So what accounts for the fact that, until recently, we ignored the evidence and continued with a habit that we knew was bad for us, and that could conceivably kill us?

Why people smoke is one of the great mysteries of the twentieth century, and a great deal of time and money is being spent trying to solve it. That's one reason why this is a very good time to give up smoking. Many old misconceptions have been disproved—for instance, the idea that people continue to smoke because they have no willpower. The complicated interaction of chemicals in the brain is now thought to be a key factor in explaining why we cannot control our seemingly uncontrollable urges.

When I first attempted to give up cigarettes about ten years ago I was told by well-wishers to eat a piece of candy every time I felt the need to smoke. One bleak January morning I quit cold turkey. I ate about thirty sourballs a day, felt incredibly depressed, and relapsed in less than three months. I also put on fifteen pounds. Are you surprised?

The shock of waking up one morning looking like the Michelin man sent me straight back to smoking. I stopped eating candy. The weight receded. I breathed a smoke-filled sigh of relief.

My second attempt to quit was after a bout of the flu five years ago. I had, or so I thought, a better handle on quitting. I resolved to live with the inevitable weight gain (about eight pounds this time). After just under a year as a nonsmoker I thought it was safe to sneak a puff or two from the cigarettes smoked by my "significant other." Every time he lit a cigarette, I took one puff. Disaster! In three weeks I was smoking a pack and a half a day and muttering defensively about it being the quality, not the quantity, of life that counted. Inside I felt awful. The years I spent training to be a dancer had, I thought, given me control over my body. The years I spent as a writer had, I thought, given me control over my mind. And yet the evidence was in. I couldn't stop smoking. Why?

I am now convinced that I failed because I did not understand the nature of my habit. I did not think of cigarettes as a drug or myself as a drug addict. I now know that nicotine is a highly addictive drug and that the psychological retraining involved in giving up a habit is every bit as arduous as the physical adjustment.

So, for my third attempt, I decided to prepare to quit smoking the way an athlete prepares for an important race—by going into training.

It occurred to me that giving up smoking should ideally be a three-stage proposition: first, a period of careful preparation to train my mind and body to accept me as a nonsmoker; second, a period of quitting during which I would learn to withstand the physical and psychological pressures of withdrawal symptoms;

and finally—and most often neglected—I needed to add to the process of quitting smoking a period of maintenance. This time I was determined to prevent relapse.

These three phases also had to be combined with preventing the other real disincentive to giving up smoking, weight gain. How could I give up nicotine without becoming addicted to food on the way?

In giving up smoking I was going against my basic instincts. I was denying myself immediate pleasure and gratification and embracing immediate physical and mental discomfort. Most of us tend to do things the other way around.

While doing research for this book I learned much about the nature of addiction and how neurochemistry in the brain can sabotage even those with the strongest motivation. The more I learned, the more metaphysical the struggle became. I began thinking in terms of "the enemy within." The pleasure centers of my brain were locked in deadly combat with my will.

It became clear that the problem of compulsive smoking was very closely linked to the problem of compulsive eating, for a variety of reasons. In fact, the whole subject of giving up a compulsive behavior is so complex and has so many different facets that it became obvious that no single solution would accomplish the task. Instead of looking for one grand single solution I found a series of smaller, diversified solutions was more likely to succeed.

It has now been sixteen months, four hours, and thirteen minutes since I quit, and I am still not smoking. So far I have not gained one pound. I believe I can say with confidence that I will never smoke again.

Even so, one needs all the help one can get. I could never have done it without the support and help of my friend and colleague Marguerite. She taught me how to eat and how to crank my body back into action. She gave me moral support when I needed it and bullied me when that was what was called for.

Just as Marguerite was my "safety net," we hope this book will be yours. Because we have been through the process of quitting ourselves, we have tried to anticipate the problems you might have and to give you ways to counteract them as they occur. Each problem has its own solution. Just knowing that someone has already felt what you are feeling can sometimes help. Four weeks from now you will be smoke-free, and as a bonus you will look and feel better, mentally and physically, than you have in years. The new skills you learn to help you deal with the stress of giving up cigarettes will serve you well long after you no longer smoke.

CAROLINE ADLER

Introduction

Stop Smoking Without Gaining Weight

> For thy sake, tobacco, I
> Would do anything but die.

Like the English writer Charles Lamb, who penned this brief verse almost 200 years ago, the two of us gave up cigarettes because of the health hazards associated with smoking.

One of us quit many years ago using a hit-or-miss method of tapering off that, after years of struggle, proved successful. The other decided around Christmas two years ago that the risks of continuing to smoke simply were no longer worth the considerable pleasure she derived from cigarettes. Having learned a few of the pitfalls during previous unsuccessful attempts to quit, and feeling determined this time to ride out even the worst withdrawal symptoms, her main concern was about gaining weight.

When we read in the Surgeon General's Report *Health Consequences of Smoking* that most people, especially women, are afraid they will gain weight if they quit smoking, we wondered just how realistic this fear might be. We certainly knew many men, as well as women, who claimed they had gained weight when they gave up smoking—and several who said they went back to smoking because of weight gain. We asked ourselves how widespread the problem really was, and what might be done to counteract weight gain associated with giving up cigarettes.

Since both of us are writers, experienced in gathering information, we decided to use our professional skills to investigate the issue. One of us would actually go through the procedure of giving up cigarettes, setting every detail of the experience down on paper, all the while reading up on what researchers had to say about the problem. Her goal was to find out how to make the process of quitting smoking as painless and permanent as possible. The other, with years of experience writing about health, food, and fitness, would see what the experts had to say about avoiding weight gain.

We proceeded to read through a great deal of scientific and popular literature looking for an overview of current thinking about smoking cessation, nutrition, and weight gain. We interviewed, both by telephone and in person, many health professionals in these fields.

The result of our research convinced us of several things. First, we learned that quitting smoking is difficult for most people, but not impossible. We also learned that understanding a little about the nature of addiction and the hold cigarettes have on the smoker helps make the habit easier to give up.

We also learned that the weight gain commonly associated with nicotine withdrawal is a fact. Most of the reports we read estimated that about a third of the smokers who give up cigarettes gain weight. A Memphis State University study conducted in 1986 by Bryant A. Stamford and colleagues found that sixty-five percent of quitting smokers will put on weight.

Even though the health hazards involved in the weight gain are insignificant compared to the risks of smoking, the fear of weight gain "was not only a major reason for self-reported relapse, particularly among women, but was a major barrier to future cessation attempts," according to the Memphis researchers.

We found that there are three dominant factors involved in weight gain associated with giving up cigarettes: a drop in the basic metabolic rate that seems to occur when nicotine is withdrawn; increased caloric intake; and insufficient physical activity to burn the number of calories consumed.

We concluded that if these three factors could be controlled, most smokers would be able to quit without the fear of excessive weight gain. The program we created, based on our personal experience and the information we gathered, worked for us. We think it will work for you, too.

1

Fear of Weight Gain— Fact or Fiction?

*F*ear of weight gain is one of the major reasons people refuse to give up their smoking habit. Tom Ferguson, a physician and medical writer, sums the situation up in his book, *The Smoker's Book of Health:* "The smokers we interviewed told us that fear of weight gain was a major barrier to quitting. Many rated it as their number-one barrier. Several flatly stated that they would not attempt to quit because of their concerns about weight gain." Virtually all health professionals studying smokers agree—the fear of weight gain is widespread.

The Reality of Weight Gain

Do people actually gain weight when they quit smoking, or is this just a myth, an old wives' tale, another justification for continuing to smoke?

As it turns out, concern about gaining weight is more than just a groundless fear—it's based on reality. Although no one knows exactly how many people put on weight when they quit smoking, most experts believe that about one-third of all ex-smokers will gain weight. Recent research indicates that the figures may be even higher: A Swiss study found that sixty-one percent of the ex-smokers surveyed gained some weight, and research conducted by the University of Tennessee suggests that sixty-five percent of all those who give up smoking can expect to put on weight.

Surprisingly enough, the weight gain itself is not what worries health-care professionals, for compared to smoking, the health dangers caused by the added weight are virtually inconsequential. By conservative estimates, the average person would have to put on at least fifty pounds before the health risks of increased weight would begin to equal the hazards of smoking, and an article in *The Canadian Nurse* states that "smoking twenty cigarettes daily is as hard on the body as being one hundred pounds overweight." Since almost no one gains one hundred pounds just because he or she quits smoking, what's all the fuss about?

The problem, according to numerous surveys, including one by the U.S. Department of Health, Education and Welfare, is that not only does fear of weight gain deter people from quitting, but when smokers do quit and notice weight gain many go back to their smoking habit. Not only would many smokers prefer to continue smoking rather than gain weight, but this government survey shows that a substantial number who have successfully given up smoking cigarettes go back because they have gained weight.

When Is Weight Gained?

Like many would-be ex-smokers, you may be harboring a secret fear that you'll end up like a guest who spent the night at the Chateau de Rambouillet in the sixteenth century and woke up in the morning too fat to fit into his clothes. In the case of the overnight guest, his hosts had sewn the seams of his clothes tighter during the night (what they wouldn't do for a joke in those days!); in your case, you worry that as soon as you stub out your last cigarette you will instantly start bulging at the seams.

It doesn't actually happen overnight, of course, but for ex-smokers who do gain weight, a change on the scales may be seen during the first three weeks after quitting, according to research sponsored by the National Institute on Drug Abuse. The study showed that even though weight gain can occur anytime during the first year off cigarettes, it almost always happens at the beginning. At six months, ex-smokers' weight tended to be the same as at the end of the year, according to this survey.

It is hard to predict how much weight the average smoker will gain. In the dozens of studies conducted over the past few years the results have been variable, ranging from five pounds for light smokers to thirty or forty pounds for heavier smokers. Jeffery T. Wack, Ph.D. and Judith Rodin, Ph.D. reported in February 1982, in an article published in the *American Journal of Clinical Nutrition,* that in comparing all these studies, the overall average weight gain appears to be about ten pounds.

Who Gains Weight?

Many factors explain why some people gain weight no matter what precautions they take. From thyroid activity to concentrations of a substance called lipoprotein lipase, the chemicals in our body play an important, if poorly understood, role in determining which of us will put on unwanted pounds when we give up cigarettes. Although it sometimes seems to be just the luck of the draw, a study conducted at the University of California, San Francisco, discovered three predictable categories of smokers who are most apt to gain weight.

HEAVY SMOKERS

Subjects who smoked fewer than ten cigarettes a day tended not to gain a significant amount of weight when they quit. Weight gain began to be noticeable in those subjects who smoked between ten and nineteen cigarettes a day. Those who had smoked over thirty cigarettes a day gained an average of ten pounds.

PEOPLE WITH A HISTORY OF WEIGHT GAIN

Weight problems are usually chronic. Those who have experienced weight gain in the past, and during previous attempts to quit smoking, are more apt to go through it again now.

RESTRAINED EATERS

There is some evidence that people who deliberately eat less than is needed to maintain body weight (probably because of social pressure to remain thin) often rely on cigarettes to control weight. Without cigarettes they are likely to gain weight.

Subjects who gained more weight during the first twenty-six weeks were less apt to have gone back to smoking at fifty-two weeks. Why? Researchers concluded that many of the people who *didn't* gain weight cut back on food too much. Since food blunts the craving for many drugs, including nicotine, those subjects who deprived themselves of food to prevent

6

weight gain inadvertently increased their craving for cigarettes. Their restrained eating increased the probability of relapse.

Why People Gain Weight

Not all the mechanisms that trigger weight gain in people giving up smoking are understood. Hormonal activity, sensory and digestive factors, and changes in the autonomic nervous system are among the many aspects of body chemistry involved. The exact nature of each of these functions is not yet completely clear.

Everyone, however, does agree that two factors are the principal causes of weight gain for quitting smokers: changes in metabolism and altered eating patterns.

METABOLISM

What causes weight gain? Or more specifically, what causes the body to put on excess fat? Described as simply as possible, any food that is not burned up by the body, or "metabolized," is converted to extra fat. For smokers, the rate at which metabolism takes place can be controlled by three different factors: the presence or absence of nicotine, the amount of food consumed, and the amount of activity performed by the body. Let's take a look at each of these processes.

Nicotine

Most researchers who have studied the effects of nicotine in the human body agree that the metabolism of smokers is higher than that of nonsmokers. In an article in *The American Journal of Clinical Nutrition*, Dr. Jeffery Wack and Dr. Judith Rodin state it emphati-

7

cally: "The evidence is quite clear that for most subjects, smoking does result in a detectable increase in metabolic rate."

Although scientists do not fully understand the reasons for these metabolic differences, they do know that giving up smoking slows metabolism. This slower metabolism means that food is not converted into energy as rapidly as before.

Food and Metabolism

The percentage of food that is converted to usable energy—energy used to carry calcium to cells, manufacture proteins, do muscular work, and so on—depends on how much food is consumed and how efficiently it is metabolized. When the amount of food consumed exceeds the body's ability to convert it to energy, the calories from this food are stored as fat. How does this affect ex-smokers? According to a 1984 article in *Clinics in Endocrinology and Metabolism,* smoking cessation brings about a 6.5% increase in food consumption and a 4.0% drop in metabolic rate. The result: about ten extra pounds.

Physical Activity and Metabolism

No magic pill has yet been invented to speed metabolism. There are certain factors that do have an effect on metabolism, such as age (our BMR, or Basic Metabolic Rate, declines with age), sex (men have a slightly higher BMR), and degree of body fat (lean muscle uses more calories than fat; a person with more muscle and less fat has a higher rate of metabolism). But these are mostly factors over which we have little control. The only reliable way to speed up metabolism (besides smoking cigarettes) is to increase our level of physical activity—in other words, to get more exercise. Almost every reputable fitness book emphasizes this point, from Jane Brody's recommendation in *Jane Brody's Nutrition Book* that "the best way to stoke your metabolic furnace is not by taking hormone pills or shots, but by stepping up your activity" to Jane Fonda's assurance in *Jane Fonda's New Workout & Weight Loss Program* that "exercise improves your metabolism while ensuring that your weight loss is from fat and not from muscle."

ALTERED EATING PATTERNS

There is one simple reason why a good many people gain weight when they quit smoking: They eat more. "Compulsive eating" was the way a Swedish study put it, while *The American Journal of Clinical Nutrition* describes it a little more delicately, saying "increased caloric consumption accounted for sixty percent of weight gained immediately following smoking cessation."

Why do quitting smokers eat more? Let's examine a few of the leading reasons.

Stress

There can be no doubt that quitting smoking causes, at least for a short while, great anxiety and distress. Stress is a prime trigger for emotional overeating. Add to this the fact that one of the main reasons people smoke is to relieve anxiety, and you can see why you might be tempted to head for the refrigerator once you no longer have nicotine to depend on.

Oral Gratification

One of the many reasons people love to smoke is that it is orally satisfying. What else is orally satisfying? That's right, *food*. In a desperate effort to satisfy the craving for something pleasurable to put in the mouth, quitting smokers turn to food.

Habit

Smoking consists of a series of rituals. We pull off the cellophane, open the package, fiddle with the cigarette, tamp it down, put it in our mouth, then fish around for a match, strike it, bring the flame to the tip of the cigarette, and inhale. Ahhh!

Food preparation and eating involve many of the same mechanisms and habits. We open the package, prepare the food for cooking, look for the right utensils, stir it up a bit, then pile it onto a dish, grab a fork, and chew. Yum!

Dr. Lynn Kozlowski, head of behavioral research on tobacco at the Addiction Research Foundation in Ontario, Canada, says in *The Good Health Magazine:* "Tobacco is a package deal. Nicotine's significant but not debilitating psychoactive effects are combined with pleasant tastes and rituals." Could anyone deny that the same pleasant tastes and rituals are equally true of eating? Some foods even contain chemicals such as tryptophan and serotonin that stimulate and tranquilize like nicotine.

The Reward System

As a smoker, you probably use cigarettes to reward yourself. Before you smoked, chances are you were rewarded with food by your parents for being a good little girl or boy. Unfortunately, they probably didn't reward you with something nutritious like carrot sticks. So now, when you're reaching for a treat after you've stopped smoking, it's likely to be ice cream or cookies you think of first. The remembered treats of your childhood may be a substantial contributor to overeating.

The Link Between Smoking and Eating

As surely as water runs downhill, smokers race through a meal to get to their cigarette. In an article for *The American Journal of Clinical Nutrition,* Doctors Jeffery Wack and Judith Rodin refer to this postprandial smoke as the "marker of meal termination."

When you quit smoking you can no longer rely on this marker to indicate to your brain and taste buds that the meal's finished. What happens? Why, you'll keep eating, of course, and eating, and eating. Without the ceremony of that cigarette to indicate that dinner is over, you won't think twice about dishing up a second helping.

Smoking to round off a meal is the most obvious and probably the most common connection between cigarettes and food. But just think for a moment of the many other ways you use cigarettes as a substitute for eating, and the ways that eating and drinking, in turn, trigger a desire for cigarettes.

Unfortunately, for most smokers, food and smoking are closely allied. Ask yourself the following questions and you'll see the connection.

- Do you crave a cigarette when you have a cup of coffee?
- Do you have a cigarette instead of a doughnut during the morning coffee break?
- Do you particularly savor that last cigarette after lunch before getting back to work?
- Do you reach for a cigarette to go with your soft drink?

- Do you light up to ward off midafternoon hunger pangs?
- Do you rely on cigarettes rather than a candy bar to see you through your evening commute?
- Do you smoke instead of nibbling on peanuts at the bar?
- Do you pass up most hors d'oeuvres at parties in favor of cigarettes?
- Do you crave a cigarette after eating bland food?
- Do you yearn for a cigarette after eating spicy food?
- Do you crave a cigarette after eating something sweet?
- Do you skip dessert in order to smoke?
- Do you smoke, instead of snack, while watching television?
- Do you find that a cigarette and a cup of coffee help you stay alert when you have to work late?
- Do you indulge in a late-night smoke instead of a midnight snack?

If you've answered yes to at least three of these questions, you get some idea of how much smoking affects your eating habits.

The tendency for most people who give up cigarettes is to nibble when they used to smoke. To have a second helping instead of lighting up. To reach for a sweet instead of a cigarette with the morning coffee break. A typical ex-smoker, as described by the American Heart Association in a pamphlet called "Weight Control Guidance in Smoking Cessation," used to hurry through dinner in order to smoke but after quitting "finishes ahead of others and consumes second helpings. He replaces after-dinner cigarettes with rich desserts."

The more aware you are of the close connection

between your eating habits and smoking patterns, the easier it will be to avoid substituting food for cigarettes. You'll be less likely to replace a "nic-fit" with a "pig-out."

In the following chapters we describe how to go about giving up smoking without gaining weight. In addition to helping you conquer some of the physical and psychological hurdles of giving up cigarettes and offering specific guidelines about diet and exercise, we'll encourage you to remain aware of the connection between the absence of cigarettes and the desire to eat. We'll remind you how easy it is to slip into the habit of substituting snacks for smokes, and we'll offer tips and suggestions of ways to avoid this habit.

2

A Three-Phase Program

Ninety percent of the people who smoke would like to quit, according to the American Lung Association. At least two thirds of all smokers have tried to quit at least once, and forty million Americans have succeeded. Quitting may be difficult, but it certainly isn't impossible!

As we've said before one of the ways that giving up smoking can be made easier is by following a specific plan of action. We all know people who have successfully given up cigarettes all at once, on the spur of the moment, but for most smokers "cold turkey" works better as holiday leftovers than as a method for quitting smoking. Therapies such as hypnosis and acupuncture are successful for some. But studies conducted all over the world show that a program that encourages unlearning smoking habits, as well as developing reasonable eating and exercise programs, is the best way to avoid the weight gain and recidivism that sabotage so many efforts to quit.

In Switzerland, for example, a smoking cessation clinic has developed a program based on behavior modification, physical fitness, and diet therapy. At the Allevard Health Resort in France, smoking cessation programs emphasize the sharing of emotional experiences about smoking dependence as well as methods of controlling weight gain. Many programs in the United States, such as the American Cancer Society's "FreshStart," also offer concrete methods for handling weight control and stress management.

The key to a successful program for giving up smoking without putting on unwanted pounds is to divide the process into three separate parts. First is a period of preparation, which we have called training, in which daily cigarette consumption is reduced. In the next week—the quitting period—all cigarettes are withdrawn, and close attention is paid to withdrawal symptoms. And finally comes the maintenance period, during which the ex-smoker learns to establish new attitudes and habits for life without cigarettes.

Training

In some ways quitting smoking is like taking an important exam or entering a sports competition. To pass an exam it is necessary to prepare beforehand by studying. Athletes train to be ready for the race or the tournament. For many of the same reasons, a period of training can help you give up smoking more successfully than if you tried to meet the challenge unprepared. A training period helps get your body into better shape to deal with the physical stress of nicotine withdrawal. It prepares you emotionally for the mental challenge of giving up your dependency on cigarettes.

Stop Smoking Without Gaining Weight sets up a three-week training period. During this time you will be told how to gradually reduce the number of cigarettes you smoke each day and how to make exercise and smart eating a part of your daily routine.

Quitting

Within hours after grinding out their last cigarette, some heavy smokers begin to experience unpleasant withdrawal symptoms. For others it may take a day or two before these symptoms appear. And of course, there are a few lucky smokers who *never* suffer from withdrawal symptoms. In a 1982 study at Columbia University, Stanley Schacter found that less than twenty percent of all light smokers (those smoking less than three quarters of a pack a day) had difficulty quitting. But the majority of people giving up smoking will experience unpleasant side effects that may last anywhere from a few days to a few weeks or even months.

The Surgeon General's report observed decreases in the quitting smoker's heart rate and diastolic blood pressure as early as six hours after withdrawal. No one can predict exactly when any individual's symptoms will begin or how long they will last, but it is generally agreed that withdrawal's most acute phase occurs during the first week. The week-long quitting period focuses on this period of intense physical and emotional stress by describing and explaining many of the symptoms ex-smokers may experience, and by suggesting ways to cope.

The *Stop Smoking Without Gaining Weight* quitting period sets up an exercise program and a nutrition program that help you avoid weight gain and keep your body healthy while it is going through the acute phase of nicotine withdrawal.

Maintenance

Many studies indicate that some degree of physiological and psychological change continues throughout the first year without cigarettes. Research shows that it takes at least a year before the cardiovascular effects of cigarette smoking are reversed. A 1984 *Journal of the American Medical Association* article found that cigarette smokers ran a risk of death from coronary heart disease fifty-nine percent higher than that of non-smokers, long time ex-smokers, or cigar or pipe smokers, but that this risk declined within one to five years after they quit smoking.

Numerous studies show that relapse occurs within the first year after giving up smoking. While most backsliding takes place during the first six months off cigarettes, it continues with "inexorable force," for the first year, in the words of a University of Wisconsin study. The Surgeon General reports that while two-thirds of the people who quit can remain off cigarettes for a short time, about half of them return to smoking after the first or second year. And it is not until after that first critical year that calorie intake and metabolism stabilize. According to "Weight Gain after Cessation of Smoking," a study published in *The Journal of the American Medical Association* in 1969, after a year of abstention, the weight and daily calorie intake of ex-smokers is quite similar to that of individuals who have never smoked.

A year may seem a long time to be conscientiously

maintaining an exercise and nutrition program, and a long time to worry about the hazards of returning to smoking. However, we believe that it takes a full year before most people can consider themselves safe from the dual dangers of going back to smoking and putting on weight. You will find that referring back to the *Stop Smoking Without Gaining Weight* maintenance guidelines on a regular basis will help you to stay fit and off cigarettes during that whole risky first year. In fact, the tips we provide for managing attitude, exercise, and diet will last a lifetime.

Putting the Program to Work

President Lincoln was once asked if he really expected to end the War Between the States during his administration.

"Can't say, sir, can't say," Lincoln responded to the question.

"But Mr. Lincoln, what do you mean to do?"

"Peg away sir, peg away. Keep pegging away."

Since there is no magic potion to make us quit smoking effortlessly, or to keep us fit and slender no matter what diet we follow, the best most of us can do to give up cigarettes without gaining weight is to "peg away."

Stop Smoking Without Gaining Weight is for those smokers willing to put time and thought into kicking their habit. Our program will make quitting far easier, but it won't do *all* the work for you. Smokers hoping for an instant cure won't find it here. The *Stop Smoking* program provides a new set of attitudes to help overcome dependence on cigarettes. The diet and exercise plans we recommend will guide you through the treacherous periods of training and quitting and will provide a framework for a lifetime as a healthy non-smoker.

Smokers who are seriously overweight, or who have other illnesses, should not embark on the *Stop Smoking Without Gaining Weight* program without checking with their doctor first. With the assistance of a knowledgeable physician they may be able to tailor the program to their own special needs.

3

Attitude

Attitude Goals

It's time to introduce you to the *Stop Smoking Without Gaining Weight* 3 × 3 program. In the last chapter we outlined the three stages of quitting: training, quitting, and maintenance. In the next three chapters we will concentrate on three main areas of simultaneous attack: attitude, exercise, and diet.

Throughout the program we have combined proven principles with many new discoveries in the fields of exercise, nutrition, and behavior modification. In the attitude part of the program you will learn to separate yourself step by step from the sights, sounds, objects, and actions that have you reaching automatically for a cigarette. Because there is nothing harder than breaking a habit, and because, like Oscar Wilde, you can resist anything except temptation, it is important to try to do as many of the attitude exercises as you can. Even if they seem childish and silly. Even if you become bored with the repetition and feel like giving up. By practicing these exercises diligently and not rushing any part of the program you will make the transition from smoker to nonsmoker gradually but permanently.

Physical Addiction

Is nicotine really an addictive drug? Yes. Although the medical community has not always recognized nicotine as an addictive drug alongside alcohol, heroin, cocaine, and amphetamines, it now does so. Dr. Jack Henningfield of the Addiction Research Center of the National Institute on Drug Abuse in Baltimore said in an article in *The New York Times* that when the first warnings about tobacco were published, more than twenty years ago, many experts thought that smoking was "no different than compulsive potato chip eating." Giving up smoking was thought to be just a matter of willpower.

A lot has changed in the last twenty years. Nicotine is now recognized as an addictive drug that profoundly affects the central nervous system.

In a pamphlet from the Department of Health and Human Services called "Why People Smoke," William Pollin, M.D., director of the National Institute on Drug Abuse, argues that the addictive nature of cigarette smoking is the primary reason why cigarette sales continue, year after year, despite the well-publicized health hazards.

Nicotine acts through specialized cell formations located in the human brain and muscle tissues. These receptors have the capacity to recognize and react to nicotine when it is present in the body. Nicotine is one of the few drugs of dependence for which specialized receptors of this kind have been identified.

The effect nicotine has on the brain and nervous system helps create dependence, which Dr. Pollin defines as "a state in which a person's free will has been compromised by the physical effects of the drug." He adds that recognizing that quitting is very difficult is not a sign of a weak and faltering will, but rather the normal response to fear of withdrawal from a highly addictive drug.

Physiological Traps

Along with the psychological factors that keep you dependent on cigarettes, there are very real physiological reasons why smokers use cigarettes to manage stress. A report that panic attacks are relieved by smoking in *The American Journal of Psychiatry* (April 1985) is supported by several studies that show that smoking relieves anxiety and that such anxiety reduction is the result of nicotine.

There are neurochemical reasons for this reaction. Nicotine contains a substance called norepinephrine that serves to counteract the natural hormone adrenaline. Adrenaline, or epinephrine, is released by the body when we feel anxious and afraid or angry and aggressive. This is the "fight or flight" syndrome. Originally it served as an alarm mechanism for our cave-dwelling ancestors. If they ran into unexpected danger, a rush of adrenaline would make them either strong enough to fight or fast enough to run away. Either way, the response to a rush of adrenaline was immediate action.

Unfortunately, danger these days comes from angry landlords, difficult bosses, a pile of unpaid bills, husbands, wives, children. Fight or flight isn't really an appropriate response. So we try to cope with the stresses of everyday living with whatever help we can get. The attitude section of the *Stop Smoking Without Gaining Weight* program will help you find new ways to deal with stress in your life without resorting to cigarettes.

How Dependent Are You?

Anyone who smokes more than fifteen cigarettes a day is defined as a heavy smoker. In the United States the *average* smoking habit is thirty-five cigarettes a day. To test the extent of your physical addiction to nicotine, compare your dependence to this definition of "physical" nicotine dependence from the 1988 *Physician's Desk Reference:*

1. Do you smoke more than fifteen cigarettes per day?
2. Do you prefer brands of cigarettes with nicotine levels of greater than 0.9 mg/cigarette?
3. Do you usually inhale the smoke frequently and deeply?
4. Do you smoke the first cigarette within thirty minutes of arising?
5. Do you find the first cigarette in the morning hardest to give up?
6. Do you smoke more frequently during the morning than the rest of the day?
7. Do you find it difficult to refrain from smoking in places where it is forbidden?
8. Do you smoke even when you are so ill you are confined to bed?

If you recognize yourself in this description, you are probably a heavy smoker and will have some difficulty dealing with withdrawal. Understanding your physical dependence now can help you with the difficult physical battle later on.

Psychological Triggers

When dealing with the problem of compulsive behavior·the urge to smoke is virtually indistinguishable from the urge to eat. One of the key "triggers" for both these urges is anxiety. Therefore, similar methods, including meditation, deep breathing, and behavior modification exercises for dealing with cravings, are equally effective in dealing with both the urge to smoke and the urge to eat.

Behavior modification exercises can isolate and control the automatic behavior that causes both smoking and overeating. It is now widely accepted that cutting yourself loose from the "habit" of smoking takes as long and is potentially as difficult as curing your physical addiction to nicotine. Just as you once learned how to smoke, you must now learn how to not smoke.

According to an article by S. R. Mlott in *The Journal of the South Carolina Medical Association,* in order to successfully break the smoking habit it is necessary to break up the "environmental cues" that prompt smoking behavior. Breaking up environmental cues is a crucial factor if you wish to stop smoking without gaining weight. During the training period of the program you get the chance to make many little adjustments in your everyday routine that will, in the end, add up to the one major adjustment of setting you free from your smoking habit.

Once you quit you will pay equal attention to where, when, and how you eat, so you will never get the chance to slip into unconscious snacking.

Smokenders, pioneers in this approach to quitting smoking, say the cigarette spends between two and a half and four hours a day in the hand and makes about three hundred trips from hand to mouth. The cigarette is also virtually inseparable from coffee, food, alcohol, and the telephone. In other words, every time you pick up the telephone you feel an overwhelming, uncontrollable urge to have a cigarette. This urge has nothing to do with your dependence on nicotine; the craving is a direct response to picking up the phone. In order to give up smoking successfully you have to unlearn this sort of automatic response.

WHAT KIND OF SMOKER ARE YOU?

Although smokers use cigarettes for every conceivable reason, an article in *The British Medical Journal* by M. A. H. Russell isolates five different types of smoker. See which one of them best describes you.

1. PSYCHOLOGICAL SMOKER
   Cigarettes make you feel more competent, more in control of the situation.
2. INDULGENT SMOKER
   Cigarettes are your reward for doing something well or your comforter when things go wrong.
3. TRANQUILIZATION SMOKER
   Cigarettes calm you down and relieve stress in anxious situations.
4. STIMULATION SMOKER
   Cigarettes perk you up and help you concentrate at work and feel more confident in social situations.
5. ADDICTIVE SMOKER
   Cigarettes calm feelings of stress caused primarily by not smoking.

Cutting Down

You'll hear people tell you that the only way to quit smoking is "cold turkey." Those who argue for the cold turkey approach say it helps to get the withdrawal period over with quickly instead of prolonging the agony. In fact the agony of cold turkey is much worse than it has to be.

By gradually cutting down your nicotine intake to ten or fewer cigarettes a day you switch categories from being a heavy smoker, who has a much harder time quitting, to being a light smoker, who statistically seems able to quit with relatively few problems.

It isn't just because heavy smokers are more heavily addicted to nicotine that they find it harder to quit, although obviously that plays a part. Heavy smokers spend a lot more time in the physical act of smoking. Many more cigarettes are lit, many more "triggers" cause the smoker to reach for a cigarette. During the training period you have a chance to gradually reduce your smoking habit until you are no longer a heavy smoker. The National Status Report to Congress brought out by the U.S. Department of Health and Human Services confirms that tapering the number of cigarettes before quitting not only reduces the probability of severe withdrawal but can permit more heavily dependent smokers to learn how to suppress smoking urges and to develop other skills that are helpful in quitting.

Each time you succeed in your efforts to cut down you reinforce your belief that you can break your smoking habit. The stronger your belief that you can quit, the more likely you are to achieve long-term success.

During the first week of training you will record

each cigarette you smoke on an index card. Not just how many, but also where, when, and why. At the end of every day you will number these cigarettes in order of importance. When you start to cut down, in week two of training, you will begin by eliminating your "least important" cigarettes. Tapering off will continue until, by the end of week three of training, you are smoking ten or fewer cigarettes a day. You will then be ready, both physically and psychologically, to quit altogether.

THE CIRCUIT BREAKERS

Teaching yourself not to do something that is habitual is difficult because you hardly realize you are doing it in the first place. If you're going to separate yourself from your smoking "triggers," you have to make some hard-and-fast rules. Think of these triggers as little mine fields planted throughout your day, ready to go off if you let down your guard. To diffuse them you have first to be able to recognize them.

Circuit Breaker I: Alcohol

Drinking alcohol not only provides a powerful trigger for smoking, it can also seriously weaken your resolve to quit. When possible, we recommend you stay away from bars and parties during the training and quitting weeks. If that seems unrealistic, here are a few things you can do to disrupt your normal drinking pattern.

1. You might want to switch to a new drink, something you've never tried before. It won't be linked to cigarettes in your mind.
2. Try a substitute "smoke," like a pretzel or swizzle stick, when you drink.

Circuit Breaker 2: Coffee

Resolve now not to smoke and drink coffee at the same time. Have one or the other, but never the two together. Permanently breaking this link during the training period will help you after you have quit. If you are someone who starts the day with a cigarette and coffee, here are a few things you can do to break the coffee connection.

1. Drink your morning coffee in a different room. If you usually have coffee in the kitchen, try a cup in the bedroom while you get dressed.
2. Wait until you get to work to have your first cup of coffee.
3. Use a different coffee mug.
4. Leave your cigarettes in another room while you are drinking coffee.

Whatever you do to break up your routine helps to break the psychological connection that links coffee and cigarettes in your mind.

Circuit Breaker 3: The Telephone

The telephone is the downfall of many a would-be ex-smoker. Many ex-smokers have reported feeling angry with anyone who telephones during the first few weeks after they quit. They are so used to chain-smoking on the phone that the effort of talking on the telephone without cigarettes is almost more than they can bear. Start now keeping smoking and the telephone separate. *Make absolutely no exceptions to this rule.* Here are a few things you can do to break the telephone–cigarette connection.

1. Keep cigarettes far away from the phone.

2. Always have something to play with, like worry beads or marbles or a pencil and paper to doodle with.
3. If it helps, chew a pencil or "smoke" a carrot stick. Anything that keeps your hands and your mouth busy will help you break the smoking habit.

Coping with Cravings

Now we come to one of the most difficult challenges of quitting smoking—coping with cravings. Because you administer the drug to yourself thirty-plus times a day (if you have an *average* habit), there are potentially thirty or more times a day when you are likely to feel an overwhelming urge to smoke. Each time you feel that overwhelming urge, the battle to stop smoking starts all over again. The trick is the old Boy Scout motto: Be prepared! The following techniques will help you through a nicotine craving. An average craving lasts about fifteen minutes. Fifteen very unpleasant minutes, to be sure, but only fifteen minutes. If you could draw a craving, it would look something like a wave. It would rise slowly, build in intensity, peak, then subside. Here are a few ways to ride the waves.

YOUR FIFTEEN-MINUTE SURVIVAL KIT

1. Deep Breathing.
Inhale deeply. Let the air fill your abdomen, chest, lungs, shoulders, and head. Hold for five counts (stop if you feel dizzy). Tip your head back. Let all the air out slowly, making a hissing sound. Repeat three times.

2. *Clench-Relax*

Start with the muscles in your face. Consciously tense them and hold for a few seconds. Now relax.

Continue through all the major muscle groups in the body: Clench-Relax, Clench-Relax, Clench-Relax. Continue down through your neck, shoulders, hands, arms, abdomen, back, and legs. With practice you can use this technique to relax quickly any time you need to, and in almost any environment.

3. *Energy Bursts*

Since anxiety occurs when more energy is being generated through arousal (fear or anger) than is being expended through activity, you can cope effectively with anxiety either by reducing your feelings of frustration and anger or by increasing your level of activity. Either method will effectively reduce the feelings of panic that had you reaching for a cigarette. So, if you're feeling tense, or you're experiencing a strong craving attack, try a quick burst of exercise. Jog on the spot or around the block. Hop on a bike, do push-ups, or twist and shout to your favorite song. After five or ten minutes of any continuous exercise the urge to smoke will pass, and you will feel calmer and more optimistic.

4. *A Mini-Vacation.*

Imagine you are on a beautiful white beach; feel the sun, warm on your body. You can hear the waves breaking softly. Your whole being feels relaxed and at peace. As you wander along the shoreline, the water laps at your feet. You feel calm and content.

THE IMPORTANCE OF DEEP BREATHING

Correct breathing is the basis of many different relaxation techniques. Proper breathing will calm you down and give you energy as well. One breathing exercise you might want to try has been successfully used by New York exercise therapist Milton Feher. Feher is a firm believer in the value of deep-breathing techniques to help people get off cigarettes. "Part of the soothing effect of cigarettes is that you breathe deeply," Feher explains. "Deep breathing relaxes muscles and relieves tension."

Most people smoking under pressure don't realize they're hunching their shoulders and tensing their muscles; inhaling on a cigarette expands your chest and presses your body down, relaxing it. You can learn to relax and breathe deeply when you quit smoking. Learning to breathe deeply relaxes muscles and lets your body sit straighter.

Milton Feher's Deep-Breathing Exercise

Use this simple two-step technique when you feel an urgent desire to smoke. For that matter, use it whenever pressure or tension overwhelms you. You can practice this anywhere—at your desk, on airplanes and buses, or at the kitchen table.

1. Put your hands, palms down, on a tabletop or chair. Press down and inhale as long as it's comfortable (count to five as you inhale).
2. Relax hands. Exhale fully, counting slowly. Repeat four times.

VISUALIZATION

Visualization is gaining popularity as a way to overcome all kinds of obstacles. In his book *Creative Visualization,* Shakti Gawain says visualization is using your imagination to create what you want in your life. If that sounds like a form of mental magic, think about how the mind can be "fooled" into negative emotions

36

by the chemical imbalance caused by addiction to substances like nicotine. Doesn't it make sense that it can also be persuaded to release chemicals that cause positive emotions by creating an "other reality" that persuades the brain to create pleasurable sensations and good feelings? For this reason, visualization is an excellent technique for coping with cravings.

Imagine Working Without Cigarettes

If you think you will find work impossible once you stop smoking, this exercise will give you the confidence you need to get the job done without smoking.

1. Find a comfortable place to sit and relax completely.
2. Close your eyes.
3. Imagine a big white ball of light hovering just in front of you. The light is shining on you, filling you with a feeling of warmth and well-being.
4. Now watch yourself performing your work efficiently and effectively without cigarettes.
5. Imagine the successful outcome of that work.
6. Hear others congratulate you for a job well done.

Always visualize in the present. What you are visualizing is happening, it isn't *about to* happen.

Visualize regularly and you will see results. You already know your mind has the power to work against you; visualization is just one of the ways your mind can work *for* you. Whatever you tell yourself, with enough conviction, you will believe, and that belief will go a long way toward making it true. This applies equally to negative and positive messages. You've heard of the self-fulfilling prophesy. If you continue to tell yourself you will succeed in giving up smoking, you will succeed. Conversely, if you tell yourself you can't make it, you don't stand a chance.

Imagine Playing Without Cigarettes

Many smokers find the prospect of facing a large social event without their cigarettes particularly daunting. Practice this visualization exercise now, before you need it. It works.

1. Think of going to a party, your first after you quit smoking.
2. Create the picture in your mind. Imagine the surroundings, the company, what you are wearing.
3. Now see yourself having fun without cigarettes. You are not nervous. You feel free and relaxed.
4. Someone comes up and offers you a cigarette; you refuse. You have the strength and the confidence to enjoy the party without smoking.

The next time you have to deal with a potentially dangerous social situation, it will be much easier for you. And the outcome of the evening will, in all likelihood, be very positive.

The Fireball

1. Imagine your craving rolling slowly toward you like a giant red fireball.
2. Picture it getting bigger and bigger as it gets nearer. Feel its heat.
3. Now stand absolutely still, unflinching.
4. Now picture the fireball passing through you, leaving you unharmed.

These exercises, used separately or in combination, will help you survive craving attacks and the feelings of anxiety that can accompany withdrawal. Practice them all during the three-week training period, and by the time you quit they will feel like old friends.

Coping with Withdrawal

To help you get through your first week of quitting you might want to plan now to take a couple of days off. If that isn't possible, warn your boss, co-workers, friends, and family that you might be uncharacteristically irritable for a week or so. If you find some withdrawal symptoms linger longer than a week, don't get discouraged. We all react differently, so remember, even though withdrawal symptoms are unpleasant while they last, they are only temporary. Armed with the breathing and visualization techniques you have just learned, you'll take them in stride.

Unless you are very unlucky, you will not experience all of the symptoms listed below. But even two or three of these symptoms when they come at the same time can disorient you and make you feel hopeless about your chances of success. Remember that as bad as you feel, you will get over the worst in a week or so. Remember also, *no violent craving for either food or nicotine will last longer than fifteen minutes.*

Continue to remind yourself why you are quitting and tell yourself often and out loud that you will succeed. Visualize yourself as a nonsmoker.

SOME COMMON WITHDRAWAL SYMPTOMS

Phlegmy cough
Don't be put off; your cough is a healthy sign. Your lungs are cleansing themselves. Your bronchial

cilia—the hairlike structures along the bronchial tubes—are lifting tar and dirt from your lungs. The process takes a while. There is, however, general agreement that in less than a year the average smoker's lungs will be restored to their former pristine healthiness.

Muscle aches and cramps

Your hormones, glands, muscles, and blood circulation will also suffer the shock of withdrawal. Soothe aching muscles in a hot bath. The warm water not only relieves aches and cramps, it's also extremely relaxing and calming to your nerves.

Constipation or diarrhea

Nicotine is often used to regulate the digestive system. Withdrawal from nicotine, a stimulant, could well send the system into temporary shock, but things should right themselves after a few days. For constipation drink a glass of water with every meal.

Headache

Severe headaches are sometimes caused by a sudden rush of blood to the brain as circulation increases, now that you're not smoking. Try a walk or a glass of water, and take whatever your doctor recommends for a headache.

Sleep disturbance

Insomnia is a common symptom of withdrawal. Try a cup of warm milk before bedtime. Sometimes the old remedies are the best. A substance in the milk called tryptophan will help calm your nerves.

Feelings of confusion and an inability to concentrate

Occasional feelings of confusion and an inability to concentrate are perfectly normal and will pass quickly. Your body chemistry is adjusting to the drop in your blood's nicotine level. The other reason you may feel lightheaded is that when you smoke you inhale carbon monoxide. Carbon monoxide robs your body of oxygen. When you quit, the brain receives more oxygen than usual, often causing dizziness.

Lack of energy

Twenty or thirty times a day you have been either pumping yourself up with an energizer or calming yourself down with a depressant. Your first cigarette of the day got you going in the morning by stimulating the central nervous system and the adrenal glands and boosting your energy. Of course, twenty minutes later you needed another jolt as your energy level fell. Once your body has recovered from the initial withdrawal from nicotine, good nutrition and exercise will give you all the energy you need.

Irritability

Apart from the effect of the drug on your nervous system, you have used cigarettes as a pacifier to control your anger. In the program we offer various suggestions for releasing frustration. Warn everyone you care about that you're going to be Attila the Hun for a week or two.

Anxiety

Although you have been using cigarettes to calm your nerves, there is some evidence that suggests that addiction to nicotine may actually produce those feelings of anxiety. Once you get through the withdrawal period you will very likely be a calmer, less anxious person.

Depression

Most people who give up smoking experience mild depression. Not only is this a physiological reaction to nicotine withdrawal, it is also symptomatic of your sense of loss.

In a few cases depression can be very severe—so debilitating that you really feel you can't cope alone. Don't be alarmed; you're not going crazy. You're kicking a deadly drug.

You probably won't experience all these symptoms, but at least be prepared to feel irritable, distracted, and generally rotten during this period. If any of these symptoms persist, consult your physician. When the going gets tough and you feel your resolve slipping, these are just a few things you should keep in mind. Remind yourself of what you'll be gaining. Your health, for one. Your skin will look younger and less wrinkled as the ill effects of smoking are reversed. Your hair will smell fragrant and enticing. So will your breath and your clothes. Your teeth will be whiter. Your friends will love you. Nonsmoking strangers will respect you. You'll be richer (cigarettes are expensive), and you'll be free of a habit that has kept you enslaved for years. At work you will be admired for your perseverance and control. At home you will be helping those you love to stay healthy. You will have taken control of your life.

—— 4 ——

Exercise

Exercise Goals

TRAINING

During the early part of the training period the goal is to get both body and mind used to exercising regularly. Exercise will leave you feeling stronger and healthier, so that by the time you give up cigarettes, nicotine withdrawal will not be a shock to your system. As you get into shape you'll feel better about yourself and will be more likely to stick to your plan. Just a few minutes a day is all it takes.

You'll begin with instructions to walk ten minutes a day. Heavy smokers may find even ten minutes of steady walking a challenge, but most will agree that this is an easy assignment—too easy, perhaps. But health experts emphasize that slow, regular exercise is best. Newspapers and magazines echo these sentiments. A June 1987 article in *Vogue* entitled "Why Walk?" claims, "Most experts now agree that the key ingredient in fitness is exercise consistency, not intensity. . . . It's far better to walk every day than to run once or twice a week."

You might be tempted, at first, to embark on a more ambitious program. We recommend you stick to the walking schedule assigned. As the program progresses the pace will gradually increase.

QUITTING

By the time you give up cigarettes in the fourth week of the program, daily walking will be part of your routine. Your exercise level will have escalated to thirty minutes of walking a day—just enough to help counteract the drop in metabolism that nicotine withdrawal promotes.

You may not feel much like exercising during the first week off cigarettes if you're suffering from withdrawal "blahs" or discomfort. Resist this urge to slack off. By releasing certain hormones, improving your oxygen supply, and relaxing tense muscles, exercise will be the very thing you need to improve both your attitude and your physical symptoms.

Three or four days after your last cigarette, when most of the nicotine and other cigarette toxins have been cleared from your body, we recommend that you add another ten minutes, to make your total walking time forty minutes a day. This isn't always easy to work into a busy schedule, but it's worth the effort. In addition to its other benefits, exercise may also strengthen your resolve not to smoke, if you're anything like a group of Swiss ex-smokers who were asked why they continued to abstain from smoking. Twenty-eight percent of them said that being in better shape for sports activities was the main factor, and ninety percent estimated their present state of physical fitness to be better than before they gave up smoking.

MAINTENANCE

Up to this point we have focused on a single form of exercise—walking. Part of the goal of the maintenance period is to encourage you to take up more vigorous forms of walking, such as healthwalking or racewalking. Ex-smokers who have reached a high level of fitness may want to begin these and other aerobic workouts to strengthen their cardiovascular output. Adding other forms of exercise, such as swimming or bicycling, to the basic walking program is a good way to keep your interest high and encourage yourself during the first year off cigarettes. Ideally, you'll continue exercising for many years to come.

There are many reasons why our program advises against vigorous forms of exercise until you have gone through several weeks without cigarettes. Unless you are very healthy, under forty, and/or were a very light smoker (fewer than ten cigarettes a day), your body needs time to recover its natural ability to absorb and distribute oxygen efficiently, a process with which smoking interfered. The heart vessel walls will begin repairing themselves right away, but the process can be slow.

How long does all this take? No one really knows. There is no sure way of determining just how much damage can be attributed to smoking. Conservative estimates figure it takes at least a year or longer for the body to recover. Many insurance companies wait at least that long before giving you reduced nonsmokers' insurance rates.

In April, 1988, *The New England Journal of Medicine* reported that a group of nurses, ages thirty to fifty-five, who smoked no more than fourteen cigarettes a day had twice the risk of suffering a stroke as their nonsmoking peers. Those nurses who smoked twenty-five cigarettes a day ran four times the risk. And when they stopped smoking it took two years for their risk level to drop to that of nonsmokers.

In other words, to be on the safe side, push your exercise level up slowly. Continue gradually building strength and endurance. By the end of the first year off cigarettes your weight and eating habits will probably be similar to those of individuals who have never smoked.

If the maintenance program is successful for you, you will probably want to make regular exercise a part of your daily routine. A survey of 16,936 Harvard alumni found that those who quit smoking and converted to a more active life vastly improved their health. The study concluded that the current exercise revolution may improve attitude, cardiovascular health, and longevity. We hope the exercise program will help you be a part of that revolution.

Why Exercise?

Exercise is your secret weapon for fighting weight gain, as well as the other unpleasant side effects of nicotine withdrawal. From the point of view of weight control, the most obvious advantage of exercise is that calories are expended during physical activity. But exercise provides special benefits for the quitting smoker.

METABOLISM

We can't say it often enough: The only sure way to raise metabolism, other than by smoking cigarettes, is by exercising. Regular exercise can raise metabolism not only during the period of exercise, but for some time afterward—possibly as long as twenty-four hours after the workout, according to Harvard University Press's *Your Good Health.*

PSYCHOLOGICAL BENEFITS

Kenneth Cooper, president of the Aerobics Center in Dallas, advocates exercise as a means of quitting smoking because of the psychological as well as the physical benefits. Exercise won't counteract the damage being done to your body while you continue to smoke, Dr. Cooper writes in his book *Running Without Fear,* but he believes it can help you kick the habit. Cooper has received hundreds of letters from former smokers telling him they would never have been able to break their habit without exercise. Regular physical activity, he concludes, "seems to have given them an overall discipline and self-confidence that they didn't have before."

THE "EXERCISE" OF SMOKING

It may sound silly at first, but the act of smoking does actually involve enough physical activity to make some researchers wonder if the *lack* of this activity when you quit helps explain why people gain weight. The American Cancer Society says that a typical two-pack-a-day smoker takes about four hundred puffs each waking day. Can all that hand and arm motion really constitute *exercise?*

It's a possibility worth considering, according to Bryant A. Stamford and his colleagues at the University of Louisville, whose study of the effects of smoking cessation on weight gain was reported in *The American Journal of Nutrition* in April, 1986. "It is possible that smokers behave differently from nonsmokers with respect to physical activity patterns that are difficult to assess and quantify," write Dr. Stamford et al., suggesting that changing position or posture more frequently or engaging in isometric contractions of various muscle groups while smoking are among the ways smokers exercise. This may not seem like much activity, Stamford admits, but "the cumulative effects over sixteen waking hours could be significant."

If, as this study indicates, the act of smoking produces enough physical activity to help keep weight down, it seems obvious that replacing what Dr. Stamford calls "mundane movement" with a deliberate exercise plan is an excellent way to fight weight gain.

BUILD MUSCLE, NOT FAT

In a smoking cessation study at the University of Louisville, the thirteen subjects who successfully quit smoking gained an average of 2.2 kilograms in forty-eight days. Ninety-six percent of the weight gained was in the form of fat, with only the remaining four percent appearing as lean tissue and water. Had the subjects undertaken an exercise program, the story might have been different. Exercise encourages production of muscle tissue rather than fat. According to the editors of Harvard University Press's *Your Good Health,* "Exercise seems to have a different effect on the amount of fat a body 'wants' to maintain."

EXERCISE AS A SUBSTITUTE FOR SMOKING

People tend to use smoking and exercise for several of the same reasons, which is one of the things that makes exercise a good substitute for smoking.

A Tranquilizer

• Smoking helps people feel calm by stimulating the production of epinephrine and other chemicals in the brain that regulate pain, stress, and anxiety.

- Exercise, often called the "natural tranquilizer," causes the body to release betadorphin, a chemical that helps reduce depression and create a sense of well-being.

A Stimulant

- Smoking stimulates certain transmitters in the brain that help produce feelings of alertness and concentration.
- Exercise increases the levels of two natural stimulants produced by the adrenal glands, epinephrine and norepinephrine.

For Weight Control

- Smoking helps keep weight down. The exact reason for this isn't entirely clear, but it is probably related to the effects of nicotine on metabolism.
- Exercise helps keep weight down by burning calories and regulating metabolism.

To Fight Boredom and Depression

- Smoking stimulates the production of chemicals that make people feel less depressed. It also provides a means of filling time. According to the American Cancer Society, a smoker keeps busy three or four hours a day with a cigarette in the mouth, hand, or ashtray.
- Exercise promotes brain chemicals that are natural antidepressants. It also helps prevent preoccupation with your own inner concerns, according to Manhattan psychiatrist Ralph Wharton, M.D. "If nothing else, you have to watch where you're going," adds Dr. Wharton, who prescribes exercise for many of his depressed patients.

Walking—The Ideal Exercise

An effective exercise program must meet several requirements. It must be easy enough for beginners to take up immediately. It should not require elaborate equipment or facilities that are out of reach (golf courses, swimming pools, and tennis courts, for example, are not readily available to everyone).

The ideal exercise should be safe and injury-free. Injuries lead to discouragement, which is a frequent excuse for abandoning a fitness program. Vigorous sports such as jogging or squash could be too stressful for cardiovascular systems that have been weakened by years of smoking. (To be on the safe side, we advise waiting six months to a year if you want to take up jogging. In any case, consult your doctor first.)

The best exercise programs should be year-round activities. Although sports such as cross-country skiing and bicycling provide an excellent workout, they require the right kind of weather to be practiced.

We recommend the oldest aerobic exercise of all: walking. Everyone knows how to do it. It doesn't require sophisticated and expensive equipment or clothes. Walking can be practiced virtually everywhere, in any weather. It is the most injury-free sport of all.

But can walking really be beneficial? You bet. Kenneth Cooper explains in his book *Running Without Fear:* "Walking may seem as though it places too little demand on your body to qualify as an effective endurance exercise, but nothing could be further from the truth." According to Cooper, "Walking ranks among the top five aerobic activities in the benefits it can produce in your body."

BENEFITS OF WALKING

Walking not only works against weight gain by burning calories and regulating metabolism, but many studies have shown that it can actually help people *lose* weight. In one such study, conducted in the 1960s by Grant Gwinup, M.D. at the University of California, Irvine, a group of overweight Californians began walking for a minimum of thirty minutes a day. They did not change their eating habits. One year later, all of the subjects had lost weight, averaging twenty-two pounds each.

At the Pritikin Longevity Center in California sixty-four patients followed a twenty-six-day program of walking twice a day for periods of thirty to forty-five minutes. Combined with the Pritikin diet (which is high in fiber and complex carbohydrates and low in fats), the walking program resulted in all of the subjects losing weight by the end of the twenty-six days. In addition, these patients, who had been previously scheduled for coronary bypass surgery by their personal physicians, had lowered their blood pressure, significantly reduced their cholesterol and triglyceride levels, and in some cases relieved their angina. A five-year follow-up survey found that those who had kept up the walking program continued to experience its benefits.

Walking strengthens and tones muscles, leading to a sleeker silhouette. "Probably more muscles are used in walking than in any other exercise," according to Gary D. Yanker, author of *The Complete Book of Exercise Walking.*

Walking is an excellent stress reliever. Unlike, say, jogging, which is not easily performed on an impromptu basis, you can walk any time you feel the tension of a cigarette or food craving coming on. When nicotine withdrawal hits, most people would find it hard to jump up from their chair and dash out to the track or tennis court. But striding up and down the hall or setting out briskly around the block is an excellent way to relax muscles, to get blood flowing to the brain and to get mood-elevating chemicals released in the body. Walking is a terrific way to distract yourself from the urge to smoke.

CLOTHES AND EQUIPMENT FOR WALKERS

One of the many advantages to walking is that all you really need in the way of equipment is a wristwatch and ordinary daytime clothes. Here are a few suggestions for the most comfortable way to dress for walking:

Headgear

A wool-knit cap in very cold weather helps keep heat in. A sun visor is useful in summer to keep sun out of your eyes and off your face; it can also be worn backward to protect the back of your neck.

Shirts

Lightweight T-shirts or sweatshirts are best. Most experienced walkers prefer cotton or wool because they "breathe" better than synthetic fabrics, keeping you cooler and drier. But some of the new synthetic materials with improved breathability have become popular. In very hot weather, for instance, tank tops made of polypropylene stay drier than cotton. Gore-Tex, usually worn as outerwear, is a comfortable fabric that repels water on the outside while allowing air to circulate on the inside.

Pants

Pants should be loose-fitting. Sweat pants or loose shorts (depending on weather) are ideal. Again, experienced walkers have traditionally found cotton or wool the most comfortable materials, but modern synthetics are gaining favor. Shiny tights made of lycra and spandex are colorful and comfortable favorites these days, although they are less than flattering on all but the shapeliest physiques. In cold weather, thermax or polypropylene blends are good insulating materials used for tights to be worn under sweatpants or Gore-Tex pants. The main thing is to avoid tight pants, such as jeans, that bind and rub.

Rain Gear

No reason not to walk when it's drizzling if you have the right clothes. Gore-Tex pants and hooded jackets keep water out but allow perspiration to evaporate fairly well. Waterproof ponchos are favored by many walkers.

Gloves and Scarves

In cold weather gloves help protect hands. Wool gloves or mittens can become uncomfortably warm if you move at a brisk pace. Lightweight cotton gloves have become popular with many walkers and runners.

A wool scarf is useful in cold weather both to keep your neck warm and to cover your nose and mouth when the temperature drops.

Socks

Orlon athletic socks are favored by many walkers and runners. Others feel that cotton keeps feet drier than synthetics and helps prevent blisters. Thick socks protect feet from shoes rubbing uncomfortably against them.

Underwear

Again, cotton is usually preferred because it allows moisture to evaporate. Full-figured women may wish to invest in an athletic bra. Sold in sporting-goods stores, these are made of breathable fabrics and are specially designed to avoid binding while providing good support against the bouncy motions of walking and other sports. Cotton underpants for both men and women are less apt to chafe and promote "prickly heat" rash than many synthetics.

Shoes

Shoes are the critical part of a walker's wardrobe, and it's worth investing in a really good pair. Bargain shoes are apt to have a skimpy toe box (the part that fits over your toes), which could lead to blisters and corns. Inexpensive shoes are often too rigid, with thin soles and ineffective treads. Unfortunately, there still are not a lot of sports shoes specially designed for walking. However, most jogging shoes are adequate for an ordinary walking program. Look for shoes without elevated heels to allow for the optimum heel-toe rocking motion of walking.

The ideal way to find the right kind of walking shoe is to go to a sporting-goods store staffed by experienced salespeople. But since this kind of service is hard to find, the following guidelines will help you find the best shoe for walking.

MATERIAL

Some walkers prefer the look and feel of lightweight leather models. Nylon mesh shoes (which are usually made with leather or polyurethane bands for stabilization and to prevent stretching) also have some advantages. Nylon mesh dries faster and is washable. It is more "breathable," more flexible, and lighter in weight.

CONSTRUCTION

Look for a padded *tongue* to prevent friction. A padded *heel counter* to prevent blisters. A well-cushioned *insole* (the part your foot rests on) and a reasonably thick *midsole* (the part between the insole and the sole) are important to absorb shock and give support. The midsole of most running shoes is made of polyurethane, although some incorporate water, gel, or air pockets. A durable *outsole* (the bottom of the shoe) that is flexible and has tread shapes for traction is also a sign of a well-made shoe.

FIT

Wear heavy cotton socks (the kind you'll want to wear when you're walking) when trying on shoes. Try on both left and right shoes. Make sure there is plenty of room to wiggle your toes. Check to see that the heel fits firmly. Walk around the store. Jump; hop up and down; rock back and forth on your heels and toes.

Do the shoes feel comfortable? Do they rub anywhere? Do they feel flexible? Never let an enthusiastic salesperson talk you into buying uncomfortable shoes with the promise that you'll soon break them in. If they don't feel good right away, chances are they never will.

Miscellaneous Gear for Walkers

SUNBLOCK

If you have fair or sensitive skin, apply sunblock to your face, neck, hands, and any other part of your body regularly exposed to the sun. Protect your lips with a sunblock stick. Sunblock will not only protect your skin from the wrinkling, discoloration, and aging brought on by exposure to sun, but it may even save your life. Melanoma, the most serious skin cancer of all, strikes about 27,000 persons a year. According to the American Cancer Society, sun exposure is a major factor in the development of melanoma and is responsible for the more than 500,000 cases of non-melanoma skin cancer and 58,000 cancer deaths each year in the United States.

WEIGHTS

Many walkers and runners like to carry hand-held weights or to strap weights around their ankles or waist. Weights help burn additional calories and build more muscle. You may want to wait until you have several weeks experience as a walker before trying this. Weights may cause sore elbows and knees, so it is best to consult your physician before trying them.

PEDOMETER

A pedometer measures your stride to tell you how far you've walked. The pedometer is not always accurate, since it is geared to the length of your stride, which changes as you walk. Pedometers do give a general idea of miles covered, and some people love them. But they certainly aren't necessary.

PULSOMETER

A pulsometer enables you to know immediately how much your heart rate increases as you walk. This device is useful for older walkers or those who have illnesses such as some of the coronary problems heavy smokers may have developed. You may wish to discuss the advisability of walking with a pulsometer with your physician.

Beginning a Walking Program

WHEN TO WALK

The time set aside for exercise is bound to be a subjective choice based on your daily routine. Whether there is any objectively "best" time to exercise is still unclear. Some research indicates that working out early in the morning, before breakfast, burns off the maximum number of calories. Other studies have found that exercise at the end of the day is most effective. At least until more conclusive data are available, decide for yourself when to exercise. Walking in the morning, before you get caught up in the day's distractions, guarantees that exercise won't get bumped out of your day. On the other hand, if your workday begins very early in the morning, you may plan to exercise at noon, or in the evening when you get home from work. (Caution: Vigorous exercise just before going to bed may leave you too charged up for sleep.)

The important thing is to schedule a regular time for exercise. If you just wait for the "right moment," chances are it won't get done.

During the training phase, the exercise period should be a nonsmoking period. Never bring your cigarettes on your walks.

HOW FAR TO WALK

You will be given instructions about how many minutes to walk each day during the training and quitting sections of the program. In the beginning, distance isn't important. How *long* you walk is what matters. Walking speeds are extremely variable; it may take your neighbor twice as long to walk a block, or a mile, as you. Your goal by the time you quit smoking is to be walking thirty minutes a day, the minimum amount of time required for cardiovascular fitness and for burning significant numbers of calories. Don't worry about how far you get.

Decide on your route before you begin walking. Check your watch when you start, walk half the amount of time scheduled for that day, then turn around and retrace your steps for the second half.

HOW FAST TO WALK

As we said before, slow and steady is the rule. While it's true that faster walking burns more calories, a longer, steady pace is more effective than a brief, rapid one. "Exercise experts have long known that the duration of a particular exercise works in conjunction with the frequency with which it is done," Gary D. Yanker explains in his book, *The Complete Book of Exercise Walking*.

When you are active, your body burns calories at a much faster rate than when you are at rest, so each time you pause during your walk the rate at which calories are being burned drops. Keep moving forward; don't stop to window-shop or bird-watch. Set a comfortable pace for yourself—fast enough to feel that you're getting a workout, but slow enough so that you don't get out of breath. Never exercise so vigorously that conversation is difficult.

WHERE TO WALK

Hiking trails, city parks, suburban walking paths, golf courses, country roads, and high school or college tracks are the usual places for walking. Shopping malls provide good, safe, year-round places to walk. In fact, mall-walking, as it is now called, has become so popular that many communities have arranged for malls to open before business hours to accommodate early-bird walkers.

Advice for Smokers Who Already Exercise

Although most smokers do not pursue a regular exercise program, you may be one of that rare breed who lights up after jogging a couple of miles. Since the metabolic consequences of smoking are far from clear, your current exercise program may not protect you from gaining weight when you quit. There is substantial evidence that the increase in body weight associated with cessation of smoking may be caused by removal of a metabolic stimulus—i.e., cigarettes. It seems likely that even the smoker who exercises could gain weight once that stimulus is removed. If you consume more calories—and especially more fats and sugar—once you quit smoking, you will surely put on weight unless you increase your exercise to burn the extra calories.

You have two choices now. The first is to wait and see if the pounds creep up when you quit. The disadvantage of this plan is that weight gain may drive you back to smoking. The second choice, the one we recommend, is the preventive one: Increase your level of exercise when you quit and minimize your chances of weight gain and relapse.

Add another ten to thirty minutes to your daily workout (start with ten minutes and work up to thirty minutes by the time you reach the quitting period). Or add the *Stop Smoking Without Gaining Weight* walking program to your daily workout. Add the walking program onto the beginning or end of your regular period of exercise, or do it separately, at another time of day.

5

Diet

Diet Goals

A recent article in the *Keio Journal of Medicine* came to a conclusion that won't surprise many former smokers: that ex-smokers have unhealthy dietary habits and tend to increase their caloric intake after giving up cigarettes. The authors recommended that nutritional education be included in any smoking cessation program.

A crash course in nutrition is a hefty challenge to undertake just when you are about to give up cigarettes. The task can be simplified by focusing on the three most important dietery changes you can make: increasing complex carbohydrate and fiber consumption, decreasing fat intake, and reducing the amount of sugar you eat. These were the three major guidelines in the landmark report published by the Senate Select Committee on Nutrition and Human Needs. The committee's dietary goals for the United States included increasing the consumption of complex carbohydrates from twenty-eight percent of our diet to forty-eight percent; reducing consumption of refined and processed sugars by forty-five percent, to account for ten percent of total caloric intake; and to reduce overall fat consumption from forty percent to thirty percent, with saturated fat no more than ten percent.

An enormous amount of dietary research in the past few years has proven that nutrition not only plays a major role in maintaining health, but that what you eat may also influence your mood. Scientists believe that messages are passed from cell to cell in the brain by electrical impulses and by chemicals called neurotransmitters. These messages directly affect our moods.

The food you eat not only influences your mood, but also affects the amount of energy you have. Whether you lead a fairly sedentary life or an active one, you get energy from food. The reason many athletes follow diets low in red meat and refined sugars and high in complex carbohydrates is that carbohydrates are readily digested by the body, providing you with immediate energy and stamina. Because they are bulky, carbohydrates also promote a feeling of fullness, helping you to cut down on the total amount of food you consume once you quit smoking.

Introducing more high-fiber carbohydrates into your own diet is an excellent way to begin a better eating program.

Complex Carbohydrates

Start improving your diet by acquainting yourself with the kind of foods that contain complex carbohydrates. As a rule of thumb, remember that carbohydrates come from vegetable rather than animal sources. Fruits, vegetables, and grains are carbohydrates. When carbohydrates have been processed and stripped of their nutritional value—sugar, white flour, white rice, for example—they are known as refined carbohydrates.

FIBER

Complex carbohydrate foods are the only sources of the plant carbohydrate we call dietary fiber. Fiber's primary value is that it pushes wastes through your digestive tract and keeps the digestive system running smoothly. But why is this of particular value to you as an ex-smoker, other than for general considerations of good health? Schnedorf and Ivy, in their study "The Effect of Tobacco Smoking on the Alimentary Canal," (published by *The Journal of the American Medical Association* in 1938) show that food moves through the alimentary tract faster in smokers than in nonsmokers. Other researchers postulate that if the rate at which food is emptied from the system is reduced when you quit smoking, extra calories are stored, thereby increasing the likelihood of weight gain.

There are many different kinds of fiber in foods; wheat and oat brans are probably the best known. Pectin, cellulose, and gums are other common forms of dietary fiber. Some fiber is water-soluble, others are insoluble. All these different kinds of fiber are nutritionally important. You can get your fiber from eating a variety of fiber-rich foods. We consider fiber supplements in capsules a questionable source of fiber, and recommend you consult your doctor before using them.

Do you think you already follow a diet high in fiber? Think again. For your intake to be within the twenty to thirty grams of dietary fiber suggested by the

National Cancer Institute you would have to be eating much more fiber than the average American woman, who consumes only about twelve grams, according to a recent USDA survey. The average man eats even less. The following chart from *Prevention* magazine will give you some helpful hints about how to put more fiber in your diet.

FIFTEEN EASY WAYS TO GET MORE FIBER

1. When you think bread, think brown. Whole-wheat (or other whole-grain) bread should be the rule, not the exception.
2. Satisfy your sweet tooth with fruit. Berries, apples, bananas, and peaches make excellent desserts.
3. Look for salad bars that offer a wide variety of fresh vegetables—not just lettuce. And make that kind of salad at home.
4. Eat high-fiber cereals regularly for breakfast.
4. Don't peel apples, pears, or peaches when you bake them.
6. Eat potatoes and other vegetables with their skins.
7. Eat vegetables that have edible stems or stalks, such as broccoli.
8. Eat fruits that have edible seeds, such as raspberries, blackberries, and strawberries.
9. Eat dried fruits, such apricots, prunes, and raisins. Fiber is more concentrated in them (but so are the calories).
10. Eat the membranes that cling to oranges and grapefruit when you peel them.
11. Snack on seeds.
12. Substitute beans for beef in chili or casseroles.
13. Munch on popcorn.

14. Add barley to vegetable soups.
15. Remember that whole grain doesn't have to mean bread or cereal. Try brown rice, corn tortillas, bulgur wheat, or whole-wheat pasta.

Fat

In addition to being America's number-one dietary health hazard, fats make you—well, fat. There is little doubt that we would all be healthier with less fat in our diet. People who give up smoking are, unfortunately, apt to eat even *more* fat to compensate for their dependence on cigarettes because fatty foods are easy to come by and immediately satisfying. Most "fast foods," for example, have a high fat content.

You may be unaware of just how much fat you actually eat. The USDA found in a nationwide survey that fat supplied an average of forty-five percent of the total calories in the diets of young and middle-aged men.

How much fat should be included in our diets? The American Heart Association and the National Academy of Sciences say no more than thirty percent, a figure many health-care professionals think is still too high. Twenty percent is better for good health, they say.

HOW TO REDUCE FAT IN YOUR DIET

With a little practice, it isn't too hard to trim some of the excess fat from our diet. Here are a few tips.

You can begin by eliminating or reducing by half some of the obvious sources of fat in your diet: butter and margarine, sour cream, salad dressings, baked goods, and other foods that are clearly high in fat. Cut down on fried foods, which are also high in fat. French fries, for example, have eight times as much fat as baked potatoes; this is a good example of how naturally low-fat foods lose nutritional value when plunged into sizzling fat.

Next, familiarize youself with the ways in which fat sneaks into your diet. The following table of comparative calories and grams of fat points out the difference in fat content of a few common foods.

CALORIES AND GRAMS OF FAT IN SOME COMMON FOODS

	Calories	Grams of fat
Bologna (4 slices)	356	32.0
White meat turkey (100 grams)	157	3.2
Pastrami (5 ounces)	495	41.5
Tuna salad (¾ cup)	290	14.4
Broiled T-bone steak (3 ounces)	276	20.9
Broiled salmon steak (3 ounces)	149	6.8
Calzone with meat and cheese (7.5 ounces)	736	37.9
Burrito with chicken and beans	236	8.1
Spaghetti with meat balls and tomato sauce	402	34.0
Spaghetti with red clam sauce	226	7.0
Pizza with pepperoni (2 slices)	440	14.0
Plain cheese pizza (2 slices)	400	8.0

Once you know that prepared lunch meats tend to be high in fat you'll be more apt to seek out low-fat meats such as turkey or chicken. When you realize that adding meat and cheese toppings to pizza, burgers, and spaghetti can double the calories and more than triple the amount of fat, you may prefer to skip the extras and order your pasta with poultry or shellfish. Understanding that baked, poached, broiled, boiled, or steamed foods are much lower in fat than fried and sautéed dishes may influence the way you cook and what you order in a restaurant.

SATURATED AND UNSATURATED FATS

"Saturated" and "unsaturated" are terms that describe the chemical composition of fats. Saturated fats have the maximum number of hydrogen atoms, with single bonds between the carbon and hydrogen atoms. Unsaturated fats are characterized by having missing hydrogen atoms; monounsaturates have one double bond between the carbon and hydrogen atoms, while polyunsaturates have two or more double bonds.

"So what?" you might justifiably grumble; "What on earth does this fatty chemistry have to do with me?" Simply put, hydrogen atoms change the character of essential fatty acids in a way that most nutritionists believe has an adverse effect on the human body. The more hydrogenated fats are, the more they raise levels of blood cholesterol. In other words, for maximum health choose polyunsaturates and monounsaturates over saturated fats.

Saturated fats are always solid. Unsaturated fats are always liquid. It is easy to remember this if you think of the difference between butter (saturated) and olive oil (unsaturated). One of the traps, however, is that unsaturated fats can be turned into solid saturates by the addition of hydrogen—margarine is a good example of this.

Saturated fat is found in animal products: butter, beef, pork, lamb, and in the fat of chicken and turkey. Polyunsaturated fat is found in vegetable oils such as soy, peanut, corn, sesame, safflower, sunflower, walnut, and hazelnut. And monounsaturated fat is found in olive, almond, avocado, and canola oils.

There are certain oils that should be viewed with a very cautious eye. Cottonseed oil, unlike other polyunsaturates, is also high in saturated fats. Palm oil and coconut oil both have significant amounts of saturated fat. These saturated fats, along with beef fat, are used abundantly in fast-food operations.

To reduce your total fat consumption to the recommended twenty percent, begin by following these nutritionists' suggestions today:

- Keep saturated fat at less than one third of your total fat consumption.
- Keep polyunsaturated fat at one third or less of your total intake.
- Use monounsaturated fat, particularly olive oil, for the rest of your fat intake.
- The word "non-dairy" on a label does not mean the ingredients are low in fat. On the contrary, these foods usually contain large amounts of palm oil and/ or coconut oil, which, unlike other vegetable oils, are one hundred percent saturated fat—the very kind you don't want in your diet. These inexpensive oils are widely used in processed foods.
- The word "light" on olive oil packages does not mean lower in calories, it means lighter in flavor. Use it if your taste buds aren't used to the stronger flavor of traditional olive oil.

Sugar

For many ex-smokers, sugar becomes as much the enemy as cigarettes. According to research, people giving up cigarettes are apt to seek out sweeter foods. In a well-known experiment conducted by Neil E. Grunberg, for example, smokers and abstaining smokers were presented with choices of sweet, bland, and salty foods. Although the two groups showed equal preferences for bland and salty foods, the abstaining group consumed more sweets than the smokers. In another laboratory study by Dr. Judith Rodin and Dr. Jeffery Wack, the subjects were found to eat more sweet foods during periods when they weren't smoking than when they did smoke. Increased sugar consumption, of course, leads to gaining weight, and weight gain can be discouraging enough to drive the ex-smoker right back to cigarettes.

The problem lies in the amount of sugar we eat—close to 130 pounds per person every year. Sugar provides a whopping number of calories that don't have a scrap of nutritional value. Sugar does provide us with energy, but you can get just as much energy from nutritionally valuable complex carbohydrates. Sugar also has a curious effect on metabolism: When you eat refined sugar, your blood sugar goes way up for a while, then drops below where it had been to begin with. The result is hunger pangs. If you eat less sugar you'll feel less hungry and be less tempted to overeat.

REDUCE SUGAR IN YOUR DIET

Cutting back on sugar will require, among other things, that you end your love affair with sweets. Jane Brody writes in *Jane Brody's Nutrition Book*, "Evidence suggests that while we have an innate preference for sweets, we spend much of our lives cultivating that preference into a passion. Some, in fact, call it an addiction, since the more sweets people eat, the more sweets people seem to want."

Like other addictions, your love for sweets can be conquered. The most obvious way to avoid overindulging in sugar is to eat fewer desserts. Cut back on candy bars, ice cream, cookies, and other high-sugar snacks. Above all, drink fewer soft drinks. Soft drinks are the single greatest contributor of sugar in our diets, with each twelve-ounce soft drink containing ten to twelve teaspoons of sugar.

Substituting artificially sweetened drinks is not, however, the answer. Even partisans of saccharin, aspartame, and other sugar substitutes don't deny that they present potential health hazards. Furthermore, the use of these substances as a means of weight control does not seem to be effective. According to a 1982 study conducted for the American Cancer Society, women who consume artificial sweeteners were more likely to gain weight than those who didn't. In addition, they gained weight faster. As an occasional beverage, soft drinks probably won't hurt you, but there's nothing to recommend them as a steady diet. For a satisfying, nonfattening drink, try mineral water, seltzer, ice water, fruit juices, and plain old tap water—which, incidentally, is the best thirst quencher of all.

Sugar-Reducing Tips

- To avoid impulse buying, don't shop when you're hungry. Don't go shopping without a list, and buy only what's on the list.
- Read labels carefully. Avoid any labels that contain

sugar, fructose, sucrose, corn syrup, or sugar by any other name.

- Substitute fresh, stewed, or baked fruit for sweetened desserts.
- Use fresh fruit purées or fruit butter instead of syrup on pancakes and waffles.
- Gradually reduce the amount of sugar you use in coffee and tea.
- Drink fruit juices instead of sweetened fruit punch or fruit "drink." Reading labels on these products makes a difference.
- When baking, reduce the amount of sugar called for by up to half. The recipes will turn out the same, just a little less sweet.
- Look for jams and jellies that have been sweetened with fruit juice concentrate instead of sugar (one tablespoon of jam contains three teaspoons of sugar).
- Eat bagels or English muffins instead of a donut or a Danish with your morning coffee.
- Use fresh fruit or berries instead of sweetened toppings on ice cream (one tablespoon of chocolate sauce contains four and a half teaspoons of sugar).
- Buy unsweetened cereal and sprinkle it with a spoonful of sugar if you want it sweetened. (Over half of the dry weight of some cereals is sugar.) Try sliced banana or raisins instead of sugar for sweetening cereal.
- Do not buy cookies, candy, cake, ice cream, potato chips, or any other high-sugar/high-fat food. If they're in the house, you'll eat them!

If you get discouraged as you try to limit sweets, just remember you're not alone. According to a 1983 Gallup Poll, six out of ten consumers changed their eating habits by consuming more fruits, vegetables, and whole grains and by decreasing sugar, animal fats and salt. Four out of ten maintained these standards when eating in restaurants.

Alcohol

If you are a regular drinker—someone who drinks any alcohol on a daily basis—we recommend cutting back during the program. We aren't suggesting that you become a teetotaler. In fact, many people find that a *moderate* amount of alcohol relieves stress. So, if you enjoy unwinding with a drink at the end of the day, go right ahead.

Alcohol does, however, present certain problems for the quitting smoker. Let's examine a few.

- Since liquor is high in calories, drinking may contribute to weight gain.
- Because alcohol is often associated with smoking, you may be tempted to light up when you have a drink.
- Drinking often clouds judgment. Alcohol may sabotage your resolve not to smoke or overeat.

Consider reducing the amount you drink by half during the training phase. Try drinking wine instead of higher-calorie hard liquor. Dilute your drink with lots of ice. Add plenty of water or seltzer to your drink. At parties, have one drink, then switch to mineral water or juice. Or start out with juice and have a single drink to wind up the evening.

Caffeine

Should you give up coffee while you're quitting smoking? Many smoking-cessation programs advise you do, based on the assumption that kicking the habit is more difficult if you can't have a cigarette to go with your coffee. If you are worried that a cup of coffee will trigger irresistible cravings for a cigarette, wean yourself from the brew during the first week of the training program. Be prepared to experience a few days of caffeine withdrawal, including headaches, fatigue, and listlessness.

There are a good many people who would as soon crawl halfway around the world on their knees as give up coffee *and* cigarettes. If you view this dual deprivation as unbearable martyrdom, you're probably better off drinking moderate amounts of coffee or tea while you quit smoking. Coffee may even help you through the process. Subjects in a study on the psychological effects of caffeine conducted at Stanford University in the 1960s by Arram Goldstein, Sophia Kaiser and colleagues used words like "active," "stimulated," "energetic," "alert," "attentive," and "observant" when describing how caffeine made them feel.

Unfortunately, they also came up with adjectives such as "nervous" and "shaky." Resist the temptation to *increase* your coffee consumption during the program. Excess caffeine will only increase nervousness, making sleeping more difficult.

Water

Nicotine is eliminated from blood and body tissue via the kidneys. During the first few days without cigarettes drink more water, seltzer, or mineral water to flush out the system and speed up detoxification. One and a half quarts of water is recommended for healthy people, but more is required during the quitting process. Drink an eight-ounce glass of water before every meal. In addition to flushing your system out, a glass of water will help you to eat less by giving the illusion of fullness. Drink another glassful at least every two hours, more often if the environment is warm. Don't rely on thirst as an indicator. Make a real effort to drink water.

Salt

We recommend reducing your salt consumption during the training and quitting sections of the program. Excess salt causes the body to retain fluid, which may slow down the detoxification process. Don't salt foods during cooking or at the table. There is some evidence that indicates smokers salt their food more than nonsmokers, perhaps because their taste buds have been dulled. After a few days without cigarettes your sense of taste will be so much sharper that you won't miss the salt.

Diet Traps

The best exercise for weight loss is to push yourself away from the table, according to the old joke. Doesn't it make sense that if you eat less, you won't put on weight when you quit smoking? Well, yes and no.

Let's look at the "yes" part first, which addresses the very simple fact that many people do indeed fall into the overeating trap when they quit smoking.

INCREASED APPETITE

Many researchers believe that one reason smokers are usually thinner than nonsmokers is that smoking suppresses the appetite. A United States Army medical research team at Fort Detrick, Maryland, in their 1982 report, "Effects of Cigarette Smoking in Body Weight, Energy Expenditure, Appetite and Endocrine Function," concluded that "the most potent mechanism for the promotion of weight gain on stopping smoking is the release of appetite from suppression." No one knows for sure why this is so, although several different researchers suggest that a smoker's sense of taste may be blunted by cigarettes. In any event, a host of similar studies confirm what most of us have always suspected: You can expect to be hungrier once you quit smoking.

Hormones undoubtedly play a large role in food and cigarette cravings. We know that nicotine stimulates the autonomic nervous system, which leads to a greater secretion of hormones called catecholamines. This secretion in turn inhibits the production of insulin. When smoking is stopped, insulin levels tend to rise, possibly accounting for increased appetite. Schnedorf and Ivy's 1938 study on "The Effect of Cigarette Smoking on the Alimentary Canal," found that "hunger contractions" of the stomach ceased after a few puffs of a cigarette. People giving up smoking may suffer food cravings because their hunger pangs are no longer being blunted by tobacco.

Whatever the cause of food cravings, being prepared can help. Stockpiling low-calorie food is one obvious and helpful approach. Sometimes just recognizing that what's *really* making you hungry is a desire to smoke is enough to curb the impulse to overeat.

SNACKING, NIBBLING, MUNCHING

The surest path to weight gain for the ex-smoker is via nibbling. All those years of hand-to-mouth activity are bound to come back to roost. This is how it will go: You're sitting at your desk, deep in thought. Your hand reaches out automatically for the pack of cigarettes— Oops! That's right, no more smoking. Back to work. But your train of thought has been broken; the hand wants *something* to put in the mouth. A cookie—yes, that sounds good. Get up, rummage around, find a bag of oatmeal cookies; oatmeal is good for you, right? Crunch, crunch, perfect. Back to work. After a moment the hand reaches automatically into the bag. Pops cookie in mouth. An hour later lunchtime rolls around. Did you really eat your way through an entire bag of cookies? You'd better believe it.

Although ex-smokers in particular have to watch out for this common pattern, compulsive munching can plague anybody, including Ann Landers. Her Waterloo was eating after dinner, when she consumed almost as many calories as she did at the dinner table. In her 1988 New Year's Day column she wrote, "I decided about five years ago that the kitchen was enemy territory, and I must consider it just as dangerous as a mine field. Accepting that single notion changed my behavior and has kept my weight stable for years."

With a little advance planning you can avoid some of these pitfalls. Since you know the danger is there, work out your defenses before you put out your last cigarette.

Think about your smoking patterns and try to predict which moments are most apt to be *your* Waterloo. While you're working? After dinner? Watching television? Driving to work?

The training and quitting sections of the program

will give you lots of specific advice about when to snack, but we won't always be able to predict where your personal enemy territory will be. Single out your potentially dangerous situations in advance and plan to arm yourself with a handy supply of slimming snacks. Shop ahead of time. Get the carrots and celery and peppers and zucchini washed, sliced, and ready to eat. Buy some small plastic bags for carrying these munchies with you.

SKIPPING MEALS

We've probably all shrugged off the "three square meals" concept as just so much old-fashioned superstition. But for the quitting smoker three or even four or five small meals, spaced throughout the day, can mean the difference between success and failure. In addition to keeping up energy levels and regulating metabolism, eating regular, nutrient-dense meals provides a steady supply of important chemicals to the brain.

Skipping meals, especially breakfast, leads to weight gain. People who don't eat in the morning are often so ravenous by midday that their willpower disappears and they'll eat anything that isn't nailed down. Another problem for meal-skippers is that dinner is not usually the meal missed. Loading up on calories at night leads to weight gain because these calories aren't burned up as fast as calories eaten earlier in the day.

Even if you're not hungry, force yourself to eat a little breakfast. Save the rest for midmorning. If you learn to start the day off with protein and fiber, you'll feel better, work better, and be less apt to gain weight.

THE SET POINT

The theory of eating less as a way to prevent weight gain gets into trouble when we consider the effects of smoking cessation on metabolism. To understand why, let's review the ways in which metabolism, smoking, and weight gain are related.

We have already seen that smokers tend to have higher metabolic rates than nonsmokers, and that when people give up cigarettes their metabolism usually drops. If, as an ex-smoker, you continue eating the same kinds of food and the same amounts as when you smoked, your body will not burn the food up quite as rapidly as before. If you succumb to the tendency to eat even *more* food, you will surely put on weight.

The logic at this point might be to go on a starvation diet, figuring that simply eating less food will cause your weight to drop, or at least remain where it is. That may work for a brief (and miserable) period of time, but your metabolism is trickier than you think. What actually happens when food intake is reduced is that your body says something like, "Hey, there's less food coming in—I don't have to work so hard!"

In other words, your metabolism drops in proportion with the amount of food consumed, a phenomenon known as the body's "set point." It's a very neat trick that has seen the human race through many famines; you'll be glad it works that way next time you're on a desert island with nothing to eat but seaweed and raw squid. In the meantime, however, if you want to lose weight, or at least not gain any more, you'll have to get your metabolism working at a rate that will prevent extra fat from piling up in the body. Reducing the amount of food you eat will merely lower the body's set point even further.

LOW-CALORIE DIETS

In addition to lowering metabolism, there are many other reasons why reduced-calorie diets are not recommended for people giving up smoking. Starvation diets as a means of weight control have been popular for so long that sometimes it's difficult to even consider other ways of monitoring our weight. But the truth is that while reduced-calorie diets may be good for quick weight loss, they aren't so good for *keeping* weight off or for preventing weight gain. Here are some of the effects people on low-calorie diets often experience:

Depression and Fatigue

Lowering the amount of food consumed leads to low glycogen levels. Glycogen, a form of carbohydrate that is stored in our muscles and liver, is burned up much faster than fat. Glycogen loss can lead to low blood-sugar levels characterized by feelings of weakness, depression, irritability, and tiredness—the very things you want to avoid when you're going through the stress of giving up cigarettes.

Bingeing

Much attention has been given recently to the connection between reduced calorie diets and bingeing, and many popular books on the subject are now available. William Bennett and Joel Gurin's *The Dieter's Dilemma* explains that periods of semistarvation are often followed by bursts of obsessive eating and sometimes even bulimia, or self-induced vomiting. This diet roller coaster is bad for your mind and your body.

Boredom

Traditional weight-loss diets tend to be boring, if not actually unpleasant. Most people have trouble sticking to them. When you give up smoking, the oral distraction of a tasty, satisfying diet can help take your mind off cigarettes.

Inconvenience

Counting calories is difficult and inconvenient for the average dieter. Learning a few basic and permanent nutrition guidelines is a healthier, more reliable approach than on-and-off calorie counting.

Failure

Finally, as almost anyone who has tried starvation diets knows, they simply don't work. Weight can be lost this way, but it is almost always regained. As Jane Fonda says in her *New Weight Loss & Workout Program,* "Starving, crash diets and subsisting on small amounts of junk food is not the way to lose weight. You will gain the pounds back as soon as you return to your normal eating habits. . . . I know. I've been there."

Eating Smart

The old cliché "You are what you eat" is particularly important for the person giving up smoking. We've discovered that reduced-calorie diets may do more harm than good. Now it's crucial to note that *what* you eat, as well as when, where, and how often you eat, greatly affects the way you feel and look while you wean yourself off cigarettes.

Learning a new way of eating takes time and effort, no doubt about it. Some substance-abuse programs even advise against trying to conquer two habits at once—"Quit smoking now, deal with overeating later" is the popular refrain. But many experts in the field are discovering that people *are* capable of working on curing two or even three bad habits at the same time. In choosing this program you have made that commitment.

REAL FOOD VERSUS PROCESSED FOOD

We believe that *real* food, eaten in reasonable amounts, is always better than manufactured food. Fresh fruits and vegetables are better than canned. Whole grains are healthier and better-tasting than refined white flour. Unrefined brown rice is more nutritious than white rice. Although there is still considerable debate, we tend to agree with the experts who think butter is healthier than margarine. Clearly, neither should be consumed in excess. The tendency today is to advise consumers to drink low-fat or skim milk, but many researchers still feel that whole milk may ultimately prove to have certain valuable nutritional properties that are lost when cream is removed. If you drink more than a glass or two of milk a day, low-fat milk is probably best. Generally speaking, though, it makes sense to enjoy a glass of whole milk and cut down on fat elsewhere in your diet. You should consult your doctor or nutritional advisor about what is best for you.

A WELL-STOCKED REFRIGERATOR

During the training and quitting periods of the program you will want to make a practice of eating smart and snacking safely. The day-to-day program recommends a variety of tasty "real" foods that are rich in nutrients and great for cravings. Familiarize yourself with the following lists of vegetables, fruits, and low-calorie snacks for future reference. You'll want to keep your refrigerator well stocked with these nutritious items!

Vegetables

Choose a different vegetable and fruit to eat each day. Select one that's a good source of vitamin A and one that's a good source of vitamin C. Fruits and vegetables have a high nutrient content and few calories.

Aspargus[1]
Bean sprouts (and other sprouts such as lentils and
    peas)
Beans, green
Beans, wax
Broccoli[3]
Cabbage
Carrots[1]
Cauliflower[2]
Celery
Cucumbers
Endive[1]
Lettuce (leaf)
Mushrooms
Onions (green onions or scallions)
Peas[1]
Peppers (green)[2]
Peppers (red)[1]
Radishes
Spinach[1]
Tomatoes[3]
Tomato juice[3]
Turnips[2]
Vegetable juice cocktail[3]
Zucchini

[1]Good source of vitamin A
[2]Good source of vitamin C
[3]Good source of vitamins A & C

ADAPTED FROM the American Heart Association's "A Guide to Losing Weight"

Fruits and Fruit Juices

Fruits and fruit juices are also terrific, "safe" snacks. Fruits and fruit juices should be unsweetened, fresh, or canned without sugar. The following servings contain about fifty calories.

Apple (1 small)
Apple juice or cider (⅓ cup)
Apricots[1] (2 medium)
Apricot juice (½ cup)
Banana (½ small)
Blackberries (½ cup)
Blueberries (½ cup)
Cantaloupe, diced[3] (½ cup)
Cherries (sour, red)[1] (10 large)
Grapefruit[2] (½ small)
Grapes (12 medium)
Honeydew melon[2] (7" diameter, ⅛ of whole)
Kiwi fruit (½ of whole)
Orange[2] (1 small)
Orange juice[2] (½ cup)
Papaya[3] (½ cup)
Peach[1] (1 medium)
Pear (1 small)
Pineapple (½ cup)
Pineapple juice (⅓ cup)
Plums (2 medium)
Prune juice (¼ cup)
Raspberries (½ cup)
Strawberries[2] (1 cup)
Tangerine[2] (1 large)
Watermelon, diced[2] (1 cup)

[1]Good source of vitamin A
[2]Good source of vitamin C
[3]Good source of vitamins A and C

Low-Calorie Treats

In addition to a good supply of fresh fruits and vegetables, several other low-calorie snacking foods can help see you through the training and quitting sections of the Program. Stock up!

- Whole-grain crackers without added sugar or oil. Read labels and choose those with the fewest ingredients (Finn Crisp, for example, lists rye flour, yeast, salt, and caraway seeds as the only ingredients.

- Rice cakes made of puffed rice, buckwheat, or other grain. These round cakes are low in calories, filling, and satisfyingly crunchy. Rice cakes are sold in health-food stories, delis, and some supermarkets.

- Yogurt. Good for occasional snacks, yogurt contains protein and calcium and is a good way (eaten in moderation) to take the edge off food and/or smoking cravings.

- Frozen yogurt. Frozen yogurt does contain sugar, so don't overindulge. It is a pleasant and refreshing way to end a meal, especially for people used to dessert or for ex-smokers craving sweets. Buy a couple of five-ounce containers and have half of one for dessert on a special occasion.

- Whole-wheat or buckwheat pancake mix. Try pancakes for an occasional breakfast treat. These mixes are as easy to make as any other mix, but since they contain whole-grain rather than all-refined flour they provide vitamins and fiber and "stick to your ribs" longer than most pancakes. Available in health-food stores and most markets.

- Bread sticks. Shaped like short, fat cigarettes, you can chew, handle, or "smoke" bread sticks. You can pick each sesame seed off and eat it individually. Bread sticks are low in calories and a great distraction for ex-smokers!

- Dried apricots, prunes and raisins. Dried fruit contains a lot of concentrated fruit sugar and isn't particularly low in calories, but it does provide a nutritious way to take the edge off cigarette and/or sugar cravings. Eat a couple of pieces for a special treat.
- Candied ginger. The sharp flavor of ginger and the sweetness of the light candying combine well to blunt appetite and mark the end of a meal. Candied ginger is sold in many markets, especially those carrying Oriental specialities.
- Sunflower seeds. Sunflower seeds are good for munching one by one. Most people find them less addictive than high-fat nuts. If you get them still in the shell, you can occupy so much time and attention cracking them and extracting the seed that you may forget all about the fact that what you'd started out wanting was a cigarette!
- Puffed dried cereal. Many nutritionists feel that puffed rice and puffed wheat cereals are so overprocessed that they've lost much of their food value. While not recommended for breakfast for this reason, puffed cereal makes a good low-calorie snack. Eat them out of your hand, like nuts.
- Popcorn. Don't put butter, oil, or salt on your popcorn. Popcorn is a very low-calorie, nutritious snack.

KITCHEN EQUIPMENT

You might want to buy some kitchen equipment for preparing nonfattening meals and snacks. None of this is required for either quitting smoking or preventing weight gain, but if you like cooking, you may be inspired by a few new pieces of equipment. Some items are expensive, but you may want to treat yourself, using some of the money you'll save by not buying cigarettes!

- A vegetable steamer.
- A nonstick pan for sautéeing foods with less butter or oil.
- A blender or food processor for making quick and nourishing soups, dips, and drinks.
- A hot-air popcorn maker.
- A juicer for turning almost any fruit into delicious, refreshing juice.
- An electric or hand-turned ice-cream maker for making quick fruit sorbets, frozen yogurt, and other low-calorie desserts.

Vitamins

Several studies described in the Surgeon General's report on smoking show that smoking lowers the blood levels of many vitamins and minerals. Levels of vitamins C, B-12, and B-6 are all reduced by smoking. Mineral loss has also been observed.

The act of quitting smoking puts the entire body, from the adrenal glands to the nervous system, under considerable stress. When a body is under stress it calls upon extra vitamins to see it through the difficult period. Since normal supplies of vitamins can be quickly depleted during periods of stress, we recommend bolstering your diet with vitamin supplements. Getting all the nutrients we need from food would be the ideal way to do it, certainly, but how many of us actually succeed? Do we have a couple of daily servings of broccoli, kale, turnip greens, or other leafy vegetables? (A small dinner salad is not enough to provide the appreciable amounts of calcium and vitamins A, C, and B-6 found in dark greens.) Do we eat a whole orange or grapefruit—every day? Do we eat brewer's yeast, liver, kidneys, or wheat germ, which are the best sources of many of the B vitamins?

Probably not. In fact, anyone routinely following today's typical fast-food diet (hamburger, soft drink, apple pie) is most likely getting less than two percent of the United States Department of Agriculture's recommended daily amount (RDA) of nutrients. Even those of us who are more conscientious about diet frequently lack the time or knowledge to eat food containing a regular, healthful supply of vitamins and minerals. Your vitamin and mineral levels will probably be too low. As a quitting smoker, you will appreciate an extra vitamin boost. We recommend taking a daily multi-vitamin and mineral supplement, along with an additional one thousand milligrams of vitamin C each day. Be sure to check with your doctor first.

Menus

During the initial phases of quitting you're apt to find that you have a one-track mind. Like Ulysses S. Grant, who turned to his neighbor at a concert and grumbled, "I only know two tunes. One is Yankee Doodle and the other isn't," you only have two habits: One is smoking and the other isn't. You'll be so busy thinking about that smoking habit during the next few weeks that planning sensible menus might seem like an overwhelming challenge. For that reason the *Stop Smoking Without Gaining Weight* program offers day-by-day menus during the training and quitting periods. The program even tells you which foods to snack on and when.

HOW TO USE THE MENUS

You'll find the menus divided into morning, midday, and evening meals rather than the usual breakfast, lunch, and dinner. Although we urge you to eat everything in each day's menu, don't feel compelled to eat it all in one sitting. There is considerable evidence that spreading a meal out over several hours helps ease hunger, prevent weight gain, increase energy, and reduce boredom.

To give you variety and flexibility we offer a choice of two menus for each meal. Every day you can look at the menus and decide which one is most convenient and appealing.

HOW THE MENUS WORK

Since the experts agree that giving up smoking is not the time to embark on a weight-loss crusade, we've designed menus to keep you energetic and healthy without drastically reducing your caloric intake. If your present eating habits lean toward high fat and calorie consumption, your weight may actually drop slightly on this program, but the goal is really to help the average, healthy person maintain a stable weight rather than lose weight.

Cooking methods used to prepare the menus generally call for poaching, baking, or broiling, procedures that require less fat than frying. None of the foods used are "fattening" per se. Red meat is occasionally suggested, but by and large the emphasis is on lower-fat fish and chicken (particularly boneless white-meat chicken breasts, which, in addition to a low fat content, have the virtue of being quick-cooking).

We have included a variety of vegetables, emphasizing particularly the super-nutritious broccoli and cabbage family. In trying to appeal to a broad range of tastes we've avoided most "exotic" vegetables under the assumption that partisans of salsify and jicama, for example, can make their own substitutions. For the same reasons, we don't include any of the more interesting grains, hoping that you'll substitute millet, barley, bulgur wheat, and the like for the more accessible brown rice or wild rice. Incidentally, if white rice is the only kind you like, go ahead and eat it. While it lacks some of the nutritive advantages of the other choices, white rice is still a reasonably healthful food.

The fact of the matter is that unlike rigorous low-calorie diets, this program encourages you to substitute reasonable foods that you enjoy and are familiar with. Just keep in mind the basic principles of sound nutrition by following a diet low in fat and sugar, high in complex carbohydrates, and with a good balance of vitamins, fiber, and other essential nutrients such as calcium. You'll be more apt to stick to the plan than if you felt trapped in an inflexible diet. Being able to choose between two menus at every meal encourages you to select foods that are adaptable to your circumstances and appeal to your taste buds. We suggest that you follow the menus closely in the beginning, but once the basic nutritional principles become familiar, go with your own tastes, using the menus and recipes as permanent guidelines to be referred to long after your smoking habit recedes into the background and a new, healthy *you* develops.

EATING OUT VERSUS HOME COOKING

For most healthy people, splurging on dinner during an occasional night out should not be the cause of dietary anxiety. If you're yearning to try the chef's special calorie-laden sauce on the main course, for heaven's sake go ahead and enjoy it. It's when you eat in restaurants on a regular basis that eating sensibly becomes harder.

The program's menus can easily be adapted by the millions of Americans who eat regularly in restaurants. Although we've provided recipes in Chapter Nine for items such as tuna salad and coleslaw for home cooks, these foods are obviously available in most restaurants. They will seldom be as low in fat and calories as if you made them at home, but you'll still be better off with a tuna sandwich from the deli than if you'd ordered a burger and fries. If the program's menu suggests green salad with vinaigrette that day, ask for a side order of salad in your restaurant, skipping the fat-laden blue cheese dressing in favor of oil and vinegar. In other words, tailor the menus as much as possible to restaurant dining, without becoming overly concerned about following instructions to the letter. By adopting a workable, nutritious plan that is *realistic* rather than extreme and difficult to follow, you'll be more apt to stick with it in the long run. Make your own lunch when you can, but when you're eating out, just relax and order foods as close to the menu plan as possible.

Here are a few general suggestions to help you to eat smart in restaurants:

Salad:
Beware of salad bars, which seem innocent enough but can in fact load you up with fat and calories via thick salad dressings. Watch out for blue cheese, Russian, and even "creamy house" dressings. Thinner vinaigrette-type dressings are better (used sparingly), or best of all oil and vinegar—a few drops of oil and a teaspoon of vinegar.

Soup:
Stick to broths or vegetable soups rather than cream-based soups.

Pasta:
When ordering pasta, select sauces based on vegetables (pasta primavera, for example) or olive oil (such as pasta with pesto) rather than creamy sauces such as fettucine Alfredo.

Main courses:
The usual rules apply; lower-fat fish and chicken are preferable to red meats. Broiled and baked foods are usually lower in fat than fried or sautéed.

Meat:
Trim off all visible fat.

Sauces:
Except for occasional splurges, ask to have rich sauces served on the side. Use only one or two tablespoonsful.

Desserts:
It's okay to splurge on a rich dessert from time to time (even better, split one between two people). On a regular basis, stick to fresh fruit salad, half a grapefruit, or melon.

PORTION SIZES

Carefully weighing and measuring portions may be useful in a weight-loss diet, but for everyday healthful eating it is neither practical nor desirable. Besides, appropriate portion sizes vary according to individual metabolism, body weight, and degree of physical activity. With a little practice you'll learn how much to serve. You may, however, find these broad guidelines helpful in determining portion sizes.

Plain vegetables and vegetable salads:
Eat unlimited amounts.

Sauces, salad dressings, gravies:
Do not exceed one or two tablespoons of sauce per meal. Sauces and dressings are high in fat, so eat sparingly.

Meat and chicken:
One quarter pound per serving is about right.

Fish:
One quarter to one half pound per serving is about right.

Rice, beans, and other complex carbohydrates:
Help yourself to one or two good serving-spoonfuls, or about one to one and a half cups, per meal.

Fresh fruit:
Eat unlimited amounts. For dried fruit, do not exceed one or two pieces per meal.

Butter:
Try to eat no more than one tablespoonful per meal.

6

The Day-to-Day Program

*T*he program starts on a Saturday and progresses on a weekly basis. When it comes time to quit, your first couple of days of withdrawal will be on the weekend, when you'll be under less pressure.

There's no point in minimizing the possible severity of withdrawal symptoms. If you think your reaction is unique, you might be tempted to let yourself off the hook by thinking, "No one could be expected to stay smoke-free feeling as bad as I feel." If it's any consolation or inspiration to you, over a million Americans quit smoking every year, and the vast majority of them spend at least one week feeling awful.

Choose the day you plan to quit. Mark it down in your Quitting Smoker's Diary. You can choose a day randomly or choose one that's important to you, like your birthday or New Year's Eve—a day you can remember and celebrate for years to come.

Once you choose the day you're going to quit, mark out the whole week in your diary. This is not the week to schedule an important meeting or take your driving test. As quitting day draws near you might find all sorts of reasons why the week you've chosen is the worst possible week to quit. Don't sabotage your resolve by planning things that might distract you.

And now, on to the program itself. There will be specific instructions for you to follow during the training and quitting periods, and two menus for you to choose from every day. Take it day by day. Expect to experience moments of discouragement, moments when your resolve is shaky. If you backslide, don't waste a lot of time agonizing over it or berating yourself—just start right back in where you left off. Remind yourself that there are forty million former smokers in the United States, and you'll soon be one of them!

Training Week One—Saturday

ATTITUDE

1. Make a shopping list. When the going gets tough, the tough go shopping! Things to buy:
   - Invest in a Quitting Smoker's Diary. A spiral notebook or three-ring binder will do. Make sure it's big enough to write in and small enough to carry with you. Or use the blank pages at the end of the book as your diary, if you prefer.
   - Find a talisman—Greek worry beads, marbles, or a smooth pebble. Buy two sets—one to keep next to the phone, the other to carry with you so that you can reach for it whenever you feel your resolve slipping.
   - Buy a hot new music tape that you can put on and jump around to when you feel the need to raise your spirits.

- Get a set of 3×5 cards to tuck into your cigarette pack to record when, where, and why you smoke each cigarette.
2. Make a list in your Quitting Smoker's Diary of the reasons you want to quit smoking. On the opposite page list the reasons you don't want to quit. Your list might look something like this:

PRO
Smoking helps me relax.
I like the taste of cigarettes.
Smoking helps me concentrate.
Smoking keeps my weight down.
CON
I hate coughing every time I laugh.
I feel guilty smoking when no one else is smoking.
Smoking is expensive.
I don't want to be controlled by cigarettes.
The new laws stop me from smoking at work.

Make the list as complete as you can. Carry it with you everywhere and refer to it often.
3. Practice the Fifteen-Minute Survival Kit exercises in Chapter Three.
4. Smoke the same number of cigarettes as usual; make no conscious effort to cut down yet.
5. Write in diary: *"Only twenty-one days till I'm a nonsmoker."*

EXERCISE
Walk for ten minutes today.

TIP _____
Remember to walk at a steady, comfortable pace, without stopping.

DIET

Chart Your Average Weight

During the last two weeks of the training period we'll give you specific menus and recipes to follow. This first week is to be used as an opportunity for charting your present weight patterns while you continue to eat more or less the way you usually do.

By weighing yourself every day and keeping a record of the results, you can determine your average weight. While we don't recommend weighing yourself every day as a normal practice, try it this week in order to chart the minor fluctuations in daily weight that we all experience and establish your average weight. Once you quit smoking, you'll be able to compare your weight then to your average weight, giving you a more exact picture of whether or not you've gained, and if so, how much.

Weigh yourself at the same time every day. Most people find the best time to do this is in the morning, before eating. Wear the same amount of clothing each time you weigh yourself (no shoes). Round off the number for easier calculations—if the scale says 126.4 pounds, write down 126 in your diary.

This first week of the training period is also a good time to add to your nutritional knowledge. Each day we'll offer culinary and dietary tips for you to use during the next few weeks. Better yet, by incorporating these suggestions into your permanent eating patterns, you can stay trim and healthy the rest of your life.

TIP _____

To reduce fat intake, trim all visible fat from steaks, chops, and roasts before cooking. Remove skin and fat from chicken.

Training Week One—Sunday

ATTITUDE

1. This exercise is designed to introduce you to your smoking habit. How many of these "reasons to smoke" apply to you? *I use cigarettes . . . .*
   To wake me up in the morning with a cup of coffee.
   To subdue my impatience waiting for the train to go to work or to get the car started in the morning.
   To subdue my impatience while sitting in a rush-hour traffic jam.
   To focus my mind when I get to work.
   To get me through an important phone call.
   To break up the routine of the day.
   To accompany my morning coffee break.
   To control my appetite.
   To mark the end of lunch.
   To give me confidence in a social situation.
   To help me relax after work.
   To keep me company while watching television.
   To relax me before I go to sleep.
2. Put a 3×5 card in your cigarette pack. Write down the time and circumstances of *every* cigarette you smoke today. Use the preceding list as a guide to record when you smoke and just what you were feeling when you felt the urge to light up.
3. Smoke the same number of cigarettes as usual.
4. At the end of the day number each cigarette in order of importance. Analyze which cigarettes you really needed and which ones you lit almost without thinking. When you start to cut down this knowl-

edge will help you decide which cigarettes to eliminate first.

5. Practice the Milton Feher deep-breathing technique in Chapter Three. Try to practice deep breathing at the same time each day. Don't smoke for half an hour before using the technique.

6. Write in diary: *"Only twenty days till I'm a nonsmoker."*

EXERCISE
Walk for ten minutes today.

TIP _____

from the American Cancer Society: "Fresh air in the lungs instead of tar will help you feel you've done a good deed for yourself."

DIET
Weigh yourself. Write down how much you weigh in your diary.

TIP _____

To reduce fat and calories when eating in restaurants, select soups that are based on broth or vegetables rather than cream-based soups. For example, minestrone is usually a better bet than cream of mushroom soup. Order pasta with sauces based on vegetables or olive oil rather than cream sauces. Pasta primavera, usually made with fresh vegetables, is better than cream-based fettucine Alfredo, for example.

Training Week One—Monday

ATTITUDE

1. Fill in your index card. Record when and why you smoke every cigarette.
2. Postpone your after-breakfast cigarette half an hour.
3. Brush teeth after breakfast to mark the end of the meal.
4. Don't smoke while talking on the phone. Keep worry beads or pebble at hand. Take a second set to work.
5. Don't smoke and drink coffee at the same time today. Substitute safe snack instead.
6. Postpone your after-lunch cigarette half an hour. Brush your teeth to mark the end of the meal.
7. At the end of the day, number the cigarettes on your index card in order of importance.
8. Write in diary: *"Only nineteen days till I'm a non-smoker."*

EXERCISE
Walk fifteen minutes today.

TIP _____
Never smoke while you're walking. Walking is one of the best ways to resist the urge to smoke, so start now to associate walking with not smoking.

TIP _____
Some health clubs can help you get started on a walking program with "treadmill walking." They'll time you while

you walk on a treadmill, check your pulse and blood pressure, and give you tips about pace and breathing.

DIET
Weigh yourself. Write down how much you weigh in your diary.

TIP
Beware the fat content of the all-American breakfast: eggs fried in grease, fatty bacon, potatoes fried in more grease, fat-laden sausages, buttered toast, cream in the coffee—it's a nutritionist's nightmare. Healthy individuals may be able to treat themselves to such things once in a while, but on a regular basis eat eggs poached, boiled, or cooked in a minimum of butter, or have oatmeal or other oil-free cereals.

Training Week One—Tuesday

ATTITUDE

1. Fill in your index card.
2. Postpone smoking half an hour after every meal. Brush teeth to mark the end of each meal.
3. Practice the visualization techniques in Chapter Three.
4. Don't smoke while talking on the telephone. Play with worry beads instead.
5. Don't smoke and drink coffee at the same time.
6. At the end of the day number the cigarettes on your index card in order of importance.
7. Write in diary: *"Only eighteen more days till I'm a nonsmoker."*

EXERCISE
Take a day off from the exercise program.

TIP
Sign up a friend to join in your walking program. Many of us are better at keeping commitments to other people than to ourselves.

DIET
Weigh yourself. Write down how much you weigh in your diary.

TIP
Sauces can contribute excessive amounts of fat to your diet. While most people can enjoy the chef's offerings as an occasional celebration, wise restaurant regulars ask for plain broiled or baked foods or request their sauces served separately. A small spoonful of Hollandaise sauce spread over poached salmon, for example, adds plenty of flavor and may be as much as seventy grams lower in fat than if the poor fish were drowning in sauce.

Training Week One—Wednesday

ATTITUDE

1. Fill in your index card.
2. Postpone smoking half an hour after each meal. Brush your teeth to mark the end of meals.
3. Practice "The Fireball" technique in Chapter Three.
4. Don't smoke while talking on the phone. Play with worry beads instead.

5. Don't smoke and drink coffee at the same time. Substitute a safe snack instead.
6. Don't smoke while watching television this evening.
7. Number cigarettes you smoked today in order of importance.
8. Write in diary: *"Only seventeen more days till I'm a nonsmoker."*

EXERCISE
Walk fifteen minutes.

TIP _____

If you have a stuffy nose, exercise may help by stimulating the production of adrenaline, a natural decongestant.

DIET
Weigh yourself. Write down how much you weigh in your diary.

TIP _____

Creative home cooks will be emulating contemporary professional chefs by cutting down on cooking fats. While they don't claim to have discarded butter and cream altogether, most well-known chefs today say they use these ingredients more subtly than ever before. It only takes a tablespoon or two of butter to add flavor to most sauces, and the same amount of heavy cream combined with chicken stock adds as much taste as a full cup of cream. Puréed vegetables are another low-fat way to add body and flavor to sauces.

Training Week One—Thursday

ATTITUDE

1. Fill in your index card.
2. Postpone smoking after meals by half an hour. Brush teeth to end meal.
3. Practice Milton Feher's deep breathing. Today combine the breathing exercise with your favorite visualization technique in Chapter Three.
4. "Don'ts" For The Day:
   Don't smoke while talking on the phone. Play with worry beads or marbles instead.
   Don't smoke and drink coffee. "Smoke" a cinnamon stick to keep your hands and mouth busy.
   Don't smoke and drink alcohol. "Smoke" a straw or chew on toothpicks.
   Don't smoke while watching television this evening.
   Don't smoke and drive. Chew sugarless gum instead.
5. Number cigarettes in order of importance.
6. Write in diary: *"Only sixteen days till I'm a non-smoker."*

EXERCISE
Walk fifteen minutes.

TIP

Instead of wearing a heavy coat in cool weather, dress in layers the way experienced walkers do. A sweatshirt or lightweight jacket can be taken off and tied around your waist if you get too warm.

DIET
Weigh yourself. Write down how much you weigh in your diary.

TIP
Contrary to popular misconception, "starchy" foods such as potatoes and dried beans are not fattening. According to the USDA, one cup of mashed potatoes (made with milk) contains approximately 135 calories and 2 grams of fat. One cup of cooked Great Northern beans has 210 calories and 1 gram of fat. Compared to some other foods—one 2.7-ounce pork chop, for example, has 305 calories and 25 grams of fat, while chicken à la king (home recipe) has 470 calories and 34 grams of fat—potatoes, grains, and legumes offer good food value for a relatively low caloric price.

Training Week One—Friday

ATTITUDE

1. Fill in your index card.
   Your new card might look something like this:
   8:00 A.M.—One half hour after breakfast.
   8:30 A.M.—Waiting for train.
   9:05 A.M.—Before starting work.
   Noon—Before lunch.
   1:30 P.M.—One half hour after lunch.
   3:15 P.M.—To relax after tense meeting. To relieve afternoon boredom.
   5:15 P.M.—Waiting for train after work.
   7:00 P.M.—To relax before dinner.
   8:30 P.M.—One half hour after dinner.

9:30 P.M.—To stop me feeling anxious while
              paying bills.
10:30 P.M.—To relax before bed.
You may be surprised to discover that without consciously cutting out one single cigarette you are
already smoking less.
2. Practice the Fifteen-Minute Survival Kit in Chapter
Three.
3. Avoid cigarettes on yesterday's "don't" list. Otherwise smoke as usual.
4. Number the cigarettes you smoked today in order
of importance.
5. Write in diary: *"Only fifteen days till I'm a nonsmoker."*
6. Reward yourself: Have dinner in a favorite restaurant. Apply the new diet guidelines you have
learned this week.

EXERCISE
Take the day off and give your body a rest.

TIP
Get yourself some headphones to wear when you walk. Lis-
tening to music encourages a more rhythmic stride and
makes the time pass more quickly. Caution: Keep volume
down. Music-deafened pedestrians have been hit by cars and
speeding bicycles.

DIET
Weigh yourself. Write down how much you weigh in
your diary.

To find out what your average weight this week has
been, add up the weight you've written down for the

past seven days. For example, your records might look something like this:

Saturday	125 pounds
Sunday	125 pounds
Monday	126 pounds
Tuesday	124 pounds
Wednesday	125 pounds
Thursday	124 pounds
Friday	126 pounds
Total	875

875 divided by 7 = 125 pounds

Don't weigh yourself again now until the quitting period is over. Getting off cigarettes is going to give you enough to think about during the next three weeks. Now that you've established your average weight you'll be able to use it as a guide during the maintenance period. By keeping up the exercise program and following the menus suggested for the training and quitting periods, you will avoid significant weight gain.

TIP _____

When planning your meals, keep these current guidelines for proper nutrition in mind. Most nutritionists recommend a diet composed of no more than 25%–35% fat (and many feel that 20% is even better), 15% protein, and the rest carbohydrates, specifically complex carbohydrates.

Training Week Two—Saturday

ATTITUDE

1. Get out all the index cards you filled in last week. It's time to cut the number of cigarettes you smoke in half. Review your cards and the cigarettes you've numbered in order of importance.
2. Divide the number of cigarettes you smoke in half and eliminate the cigarettes on the bottom half of the list from your life. Yup, just like that. Those butts are history!
3. Make a list of when you wish to smoke the cigarettes in the top half of your list. Once you have made the list, stick to it. Smoke only according to your schedule. *Try not to cheat.* If you decide on ten, stick to ten. Don't have an extra cigarette in the morning and tell yourself you'll make up for it in the afternoon. You won't. Cheating is habit-forming. Control and nicotine reduction are the point here. *Stick to your schedule.*

   Here's a sample list of the way you might plan your smoking schedule. Change it to suit your needs. But remember, stick to the smoking plan you decide on.

   1   Half an hour after breakfast.
   1   Before starting work.
   1   Half an hour after coffee break.
   1   Half an hour after lunch.
   1   Before starting work after lunch.
   1   Midafternoon.
   1   Immediately after work.
   1   Half an hour before dinner.
   1   Half an hour after dinner.

1 Later in the evening.
1 Before bed.

4 Remember your list of pros and cons? It's time for an update. Have your feelings about smoking changed? Don't leave home without your list; consult it often.

5. Use breathing techniques and visualization to get through cravings. Practice your Fifteen-Minute Survival Kit.

6. Record the times your urge to smoke is most severe in your diary. Tomorrow you can try to avoid those situations.

7. Write in diary: *"Only Fourteen days till I'm a non-smoker."*

8. Reward yourself: Make an appointment to have a full-body massage, or plan dinner in a favorite restaurant. Find a different way to reward yourself every day this week. For years you have been rewarding yourself with cigarettes; think of all the fun you've been missing!

TIP

Be realistic in the goals you set. If you decide to smoke one cigarette an hour, that's a realistic goal. Make a schedule you can stick to.

EXERCISE
Walk fifteen minutes.

TIP

Make a conscious effort to swing your arms while you walk.

TIP

Mark the end of your first week's exercise program with a small reward. Buy yourself a colorful pair of walking socks, knit gloves, or a cool tank top if the weather is warm. Or get a lightweight backpack, "fanny-pack," or small pack that fits around your waist for carrying your wallet, keys, etc. Sporting-goods stores also sell small carriers that you attach to your shoe.

DIET

Morning
1.
½ papaya
1 glass orange juice
1 toasted English muffin or bagel spread with cottage
    cheese or peanut butter

Snack: 1 rice cake

or

2.
1 orange, peeled and thinly sliced
1 scrambled egg, preferably cooked without butter in
    nonstick pan
1 piece whole-grain toast

Snack: any amount your choice raw vegetables

Midday
1.
Salade Niçoise*
2–4 whole-grain crackers
Sliced berries

Snack: One glass grape juice, 3 bread sticks

or

2.
Crab Melt*
1 tomato, cut in wedges

Snack: 1 fresh pear or peach

TIP _____

Most cheese is high in fat and calories. An ounce of cheddar has about 115 calories and 9.4 grams of fat, and an ounce of Swiss has 107 calories and 7.8 grams of fat. "Manufactured" cheeses are no better than natural ones: one ounce American cheese contains 106 calories and 7.8 grams fat. Your best bets are cottage cheese (2% fat), with 25 calories per ounce and .5 gram fat, ricotta (39 calories, 2.2 grams fat), part-skim mozzarella (72 calories, 4.5 grams fat), and feta, with 75 calories and 6.0 grams fat (but be aware that feta is high in salt).

_____

Evening
1.
Chicken with Chilies*
Orzo Baked with Garlic and Cheese*
Steamed broccoli drizzled with olive oil and lemon
     juice, served cold or warm
Cold Coffee Soufflé*

Snack: popcorn (no oil or butter)

or

2.

Treat yourself to dinner at your favorite Mexican
restaurant.
6 tortilla chips with salsa
1 chicken or bean tostada
Fresh fruit in season, any amount

Snack: 4 bread sticks

TIP _____

from the American Heart Association: Eat something low-
calorie before you go to a party so you won't face a tableful of
appetizers on an empty stomach. Do your "mingling" away
from the table.

TIP _____

By stimulating taste buds, spicy foods can help alleviate
nicotine cravings.

Training Week Two—Sunday

ATTITUDE

1. Smoke cigarettes according to schedule. You
   should be smoking no more than fifteen cigarettes
   per day.
2. Use deep breathing, visualization, and Fifteen-Minute Survival Kit to get through cravings.
3. Avoid bars and other smoky places. You're only
   human. Breathing the air in those places can be like
   smoking a cigarette.

4. Consciously avoid at least one of the difficult "urge" situations you recorded in your diary yesterday.
5. Seek out nonsmoking situations. Ask for nonsmoking seats in restaurants and other public places. Practice thinking of yourself as a nonsmoker.
6. Write in diary: *"Only thirteen days till I'm a nonsmoker."*
7. Reward yourself: Go to a movie or concert.

EXERCISE
Walk fifteen minutes.

TIP
While you swing your arms rhythmically with each step, also concentrate on lengthening your stride. Long strides and a vigorous arm swing add to a workout by burning more calories.

DIET

Morning
1.
½ grapefruit
1 poached egg on whole-wheat toast

Snack: 1 tangerine

or

2.
Fresh pineapple chunks
2 small or 1 large bran muffin, preferable Blueberry Bran Muffins*

Snack: 1 "Smoothie"*—flavor of your choice

Midday
1.
1 bowl Broccoli Soup*
2–4 whole grain crackers
1 cup unflavored or vanilla yogurt with 1 sliced
      banana

Snack: Any amount carrot sticks with Low-Fat Dip,*
flavor of your choice

or

2.
Chicken Salad* sandwich on whole-grain or whole-
      wheat bread with lettuce and tomato
1 bowl fresh strawberries or raspberries

Snack: 1 glass low-fat milk.

TIP _____

from the American Heart Association: "Eating a variety of
foods is essential to get all the nutrients you need."

Evening
1.
3 to 5 ounces broiled sole or flounder garnished with
      lemon wedges
1 baked potato, preferably topped with yogurt and
      green onions
Raw spinach salad with Vinaigrette*
Angel Food Cake* with fresh berries

Snack: 1 tangerine

119

or

2.
Baked Salmon with Capers*
New Potatoes Roasted with Garlic and Rosemary*
Mixed green salad with Vinaigrette*
1 bowl fresh pineapple chunks mixed with berries
2 oatmeal cookies

Snack: 1 rice cake

Training Week Two—Monday

ATTITUDE

1. Smoke cigarettes according to schedule.
2. Use deep breathing, visualization, and Fifteen-Minute Survival Kit to get through cravings.
3. Avoid smoky places and smoking people.
4. Write in diary: *"Only twelve days till I'm a nonsmoker."*
5. Reward yourself: Have your hair done or have a shave at a barber shop.

EXERCISE
Walk twenty minutes.

TIP
from the American Cancer Society: "Exercise is a great substitute for smoking. A body that is pleasantly tired from exertion is less likely to want a cigarette."

DIET

Morning
1.
1 orange, whole or freshly squeezed juice
1 bowl sliced berries with milk
2 small or 1 large bran muffin, preferable Blueberry
    Bran Muffins*

Snack: 1 glass low-fat milk

or

2.
½ grapefruit
1 bowl dry cereal with strawberries or ½ banana
1 piece whole-grain toast

Snack: 1 glass V-8 or tomato juice

Midday
1.
1 Turkey Salad* sandwich on whole-grain bread with
    lettuce and tomato
Coleslaw*
1 tangerine

or

2.
Cottage cheese with fresh pineapple chunks or other
    fruit
2 rice cakes

Snack: 6–8 broccoli flowerets or one wedge raw cabbage with Low-Fat Dip,* your choice of flavor.

TIP _____

Sip instead of puff. Drink your juice and other beverages slowly. If you make them last, the urge to smoke will pass.

Evening

1.
3 to 5-ounce broiled pork chop
Lima Beans with Garlic*
Mixed green salad, oil and vinegar
1 baked apple

Snack: 1 glass grape juice and a handful of sunflower seeds (about ⅓ cup)

or

2.
Crab Bisque*
Chicken Breasts with Fresh Coriander Sauce*
Rice, preferably brown
2 or 3 sliced tomatoes with minced fresh herbs
2 oatmeal cookies or strawberry frozen yogurt (no more than ½ cup)

Snack: Sliced banana with ½ cup low-fat milk

Training Week Two—Tuesday

ATTITUDE

1. Plan to smoke no more than fourteen cigarettes today. Cross your "least important" cigarettes off your list. If you are already smoking fewer than fourteen cigarettes, eliminate one more.
2. Use deep breathing and visualization techniques and the Fifteen-Minute Survival Kit to get through cravings.
3. Carry your talisman with you. Play with your pebble or worry beads whenever you feel yourself getting tense. It will relax you.
4. Consult your pros and cons list and remind yourself why you started the program.
5. Write in diary: *"Only eleven days till I'm a non-smoker."*
6. Reward yourself: Buy yourself a small present. A pair of red socks or a grown-up toy.

EXERCISE
Take the day off.

DIET

Morning
1.
½ papaya
1 bowl dry cereal with milk and 1 banana
1 piece whole-grain toast

Snack: ⅓ cup raisins

or

2.
½ cantaloupe or other melon
1 bowl oatmeal or other hot cereal
1 piece whole-grain toast

Snack: Small bunch grapes and 5–6 melon cubes

TIP _____

Instead of sweetening oatmeal or other hot cereal with sugar, try a handful of raisins or sliced banana.

Midday
1.
1 cup Broccoli Soup,* served cold and topped with a
    spoonful of unflavored yogurt
1 toasted bagel or English muffin sprinkled with
    parmesan
1 baked apple

Snack: 8–10 raw green beans or sugar peas, 6 carrot sticks.

or

2.
Salmon Salad* served on lettuce leaves, garnished
    with tomato wedges and sliced cucumber
2–4 whole-grain crackers
1 fresh nectarine or pear

Snack: V-8 or tomato juice

Evening

1.

1 cup Cherry Tomato Soup*

1 cup Eggplant Pudding*

Steamed brussels sprouts seasoned with lemon juice
and dill

Raw carrot sticks

Frozen raspberry yogurt (no more than ½ cup)

Snack: 4 bread sticks

or

2.

1 small grilled steak

1 cup mashed potatoes

1 cup steamed carrots

Mixed green salad

1 wedge honeydew melon or watermelon

Snack: small bunch grapes

TIP _____

For variety and convenience, make double portions of soup.
Serve half hot one night and the rest cold later in the week.

Training Week Two—Wednesday

ATTITUDE

1. Plan to smoke no more than thirteen cigarettes today. If you're already below thirteen, cross your "least important" cigarette off your list.
2. Use deep breathing and visualization techniques and Fifteen-Minute Survival Kit to get through cravings.
3. "Smoke" straws and cinnamon sticks. Don't forget your talisman. Your hands and your mouth are used to being kept busy with smoking. Keep them busy doing these other, nonfattening things.
4. Write in diary: *"Only ten days till I'm a nonsmoker."*
5. Reward yourself: Join the local library or gym.

EXERCISE
Walk twenty minutes.

TIP

The first few minutes of a workout can be boring, tiring, and a nuisance. Experienced exercisers know that these feelings usually pass. Don't get discouraged. Stick with your walking for the full twenty minutes.

DIET

Morning
1.
½ grapefruit
1 bowl oatmeal or other whole-grain hot cereal
½ English muffin

Snack: 1 serving yogurt, preferably unsweetened

or

2.
½ grapefruit
1 poached egg on 1 piece whole-grain toast

Snack: One glass apple juice

Midday
1.
One 1-egg mushroom omelette
1 tomato, sliced
1 kiwi or fresh plum
2 Gingerbread Crisps* or gingersnaps

Snack: 1 apple

or

2.
1 cheese sandwich, broiled, on English muffin or rye
    bread, with mozzarella and sliced fresh tomato
1 cup applesauce

Snack: 6–8 broccoli or cauliflower flowerettes

TIP

Drink water with your snack, before meals, and once or twice during the morning and afternoon. Even if you haven't been a water drinker in the past, you'll feel better and less hungry when you're properly hydrated.

Evening

1.
Steamed Mussels in White Wine*
Mixed green salad with Vinaigrette*
Chocolate Sponge Cake* or sliced fresh peaches

Snack: 1 glass orange juice or orange spritzer (orange juice with a splash of seltzer)

or

2.
Artichokes with Yogurt Sauce Verte*
Chicken with Chilies*
1 baked potato
1 cup fresh fruit salad

Snack: 1 whole-grain cracker spread with cottage cheese

Training Week Two—Thursday

ATTITUDE

1. Plan to smoke no more than twelve cigarettes today, or one less than yesterday's total if you're below twelve.
   By now you are down to your "important" cigarettes. Eliminate one cigarette after lunch today.
2. Use deep breathing and visualization techniques and the Fifteen-Minute Survival Kit to get through cravings.
3. Avoid all the "Don'ts" on last Thursday's list.
4. Write in your diary: *"Only nine days till I'm a nonsmoker."*

5. Reward yourself: Take a boat ride or have a picnic.

EXERCISE
Walk twenty minutes.

TIP _____

Many women are afraid that exercising will "build big, ugly muscles." A walking program will strengthen and tone muscles but will not "pump them up."

DIET

Morning

1. orange (whole or fresh-squeezed juice)
2. slices whole-grain French toast, preferably topped with fruit styrup and unflavored yogurt; use maple syrup sparingly

Snack: 1 small handful sunflower seeds (about ⅓ cup)

or

2.

1. tangerine
2. serving yogurt, preferably unsweetened, topped with fresh berries, ½ banana, sliced, and 1 teaspoon wheat germ (optional)

Snack: ½ bagel, preferably plain but with no more than teaspoon butter or cream cheese

TIP _____

from the American Heart Association: "It's not unusual for family members or friends, however well-intentioned, to undermine your diet. Be polite but firm, and don't back down. You don't have to explain or apologize."

Midday

1.
1 Chicken Salad* sandwich on whole-grain bread
    with lettuce and tomato
½ cantaloupe

Snack: Any amount of raw vegetables

or

2.
1 cup chili beans
1 small salad, lettuce and tomato, with Vinaigrette*

Snack: 1 glass apple juice.

TIP _____

The cookie jar is a symbol of childhood happiness in America. If you can't do without these sweet treats, consider this: According to a recent survey conducted by Laurie Quint of the Center for Science in the Public Interest, most cookies derive 40% of their calories from fat and another 30% from sugar. The best low-fat cookies are graham crackers and gingersnaps, which have less than 1 teaspoon of fat per 1-ounce serving (2–3 cookies). Oatmeal cookies contain some fat, but also moderate amounts of fiber. Use cookies as occasional "rewards," but don't let your sweet tooth get the best of you.

Evening

1.
Baked Salmon with Capers*
Wild rice or brown rice
Steamed broccoli seasoned with lemon juice
Mixed fruit salad
2 Gingerbread Crisps* or gingersnaps

Snack: 1 glass grapefruit juice

or

2.
Spaghetti with Fresh Tomato Sauce*
Mixed green salad with Vinaigrette*
8 strawberries sprinkled with lemon juice and ½
    teaspoon sugar

Snack: 1 apple

Training Week Two—Friday

ATTITUDE

1. Plan to smoke no more than eleven cigarettes today
   (if you're below eleven, eliminate one more).
2. Review pro and con list. Alter it to reflect your
   changing attitude toward smoking.
3. Take a few moments to think about your successes
   this week:
   • You have greatly reduced your smoking habit.
   • You have improved the way you eat and exercise.
   • You have learned new skills to help you manage
     anxiety and stress.

Congratulations!
4. Give yourself a firm pat on the back. You deserve it!
5. Write in your diary: *"Only eight days till I'm a nonsmoker."*
6. Reward yourself: Buy some exotic fruits and vegetables at your local market.

EXERCISE
Walk twenty minutes.

TIP _____
There are lots of other walkers out there. Fifty-five million Americans list walking as their favorite form of exercise.

DIET

Morning
1.
1 cup fresh pineapple chunks
1 bowl oatmeal or other whole-grain hot cereal
1 slice whole-grain toast

Snack: 1 serving yogurt, preferably unsweetened

or

2.
1 whole orange or orange juice
1-egg mushroom omelette
1 slice whole-grain toast

Snack: 1 small bunch grapes

Midday

1.
1 bowl lentil soup
1 mixed green salad with Vinaigrette*
2–4 rice cakes or whole-grain crackers

Snack: 4 1-inch cubes mozzarella cheese, one glass apple juice.

or

2.
½ avocado stuffed with Tuna Salad*
5 cherry tomatoes
2–4 whole-grain crackers

Snack: 1 glass orange juice or orange spritzer (orange juice with a splash of seltzer)

Evening

1.
Broiled or grilled chicken kabobs (skewered with
    chunks of green pepper, onion, mushroom, and
    cherry tomatoes)
Steamed broccoli
Brown rice or wild rice
Chocolate Sponge Cake* or 2 oatmeal cookies

Snack: 4 bread sticks

or

2.
1 3- to 5-ounce lamb chop (fat trimmed off), broiled
1 baked potato

Steamed green beans
Coleslaw*
Baked apple

Snack: 1 rice cake

Training Week Three—Saturday

THE FINAL COUNTDOWN

You're getting pretty good at this. You might be feeling so confident that you're tempted to skip the next week of training and advance straight to quitting. Don't do it! As you've no doubt realized, quitting is not just a question of getting through withdrawal symptoms. You are also giving up a firmly entrenched habit. When you give up smoking without addressing both problems you risk relapse.

According to the 1986 National Status Report on Smoking and Health, 70%–80% of quitters relapse in the first year. The majority of people who do quit for good have tried giving up before and failed. If you follow the *Stop Smoking Without Gaining Weight* program to its conclusion, you will avoid the many pitfalls that can cause relapse. The three-week training period is an essential part of "letting go." Keep up the good work!

ATTITUDE

1. Cut cigarettes to no more than ten a day. If you're already down to less than ten a day, stay where you are. Ten or fewer cigarettes a day put you in the "light smoker" category. (Remember, light smokers are the ones that have less trouble quitting.) You

won't have to cut down anymore until Quitting-Day. Once you are comfortable with your firmly scheduled ten cigarettes a day, you are ready to quit. Make your schedule for when to smoke your ten, and stick to it. If you try to decide which cigarettes are important on an ad hoc basis, you're making things too tough on yourself. When you really crave a cigarette, they're *all* equally important!

2. Seek out situations where you can't smoke. Avoid smoke-filled bars this evening. Go to a movie. Sit in the nonsmoking section of a restaurant.

3. Record in your diary how your feelings about smoking have changed. Write down when you find not smoking the most difficult.

4. Write in diary: *"Only seven days till I'm a nonsmoker."*

5. Reward yourself: Buy a magazine you've never read.

EXERCISE
Walk twenty minutes.

TIP _____

Think you're too old to follow a regular exercise program? George Sheehan and Bob Holtel wouldn't agree. Writer and champion runner Sheehan didn't start running until he was forty-five. He is still training and racing regularly at age sixty-nine. Fifty-six year old Holtel spent the last three summers running the length of the Pacific Crest Trail, a total of 2,581 miles from the Mexican to Canadian borders. "I'm proud and satisfied that I completed it," he said in a 1988 interview in *Runner's World*. "I still run eighty miles a week whether I'm going to Canada or not."

DIET

Morning
1.
½ grapefruit
1 soft-boiled or poached egg
1 slice whole-grain toast

Snack: apple juice

or

2.
Whole-wheat or buckwheat pancakes, preferably with
     pure maple syrup or fruit syrup
Fresh blueberries or strawberries

Snack: 1 glass low-fat milk

TIP _____
Try yogurt instead of butter on pancakes or waffles for a
tasty, low-fat treat.

TIP _____
Canadian bacon contains less fat than regular bacon.

Midday
1.
"Smoothie"*—flavor of your choice
2–4 whole-grain crackers or rice cakes
½ cantaloupe

Snack: 5 strawberries or 1 mango

or

2.
1 bowl tomato soup or Cherry Tomato Soup*
1 English muffin; top with ricotta or cottage cheese
    and broil
1 cup applesauce, preferably unsweetened
2 Gingerbread Crisps* or gingersnaps

Snack: any amount of raw vegetables

TIP _____

from the American Lung Association: "For weight control,
use smaller plates and bowls to give the impression of more
food. Chew slowly. Rest your fork and knife between bites.
Give your body twenty minutes to digest the meal and tell
you it's satisfied."

Evening
1.
Crab Bisque*
Chicken Marinated with Oregano*
Corn on the cob or peas
Coleslaw*
Poached Peaches in Red Wine and Honey* or sliced
    fresh mango

Snack: 1 rice cake

or

2.
Treat yourself to dinner at your favorite Italian
    restaurant.

1 cup minestrone soup
Mixed green salad, oil and vinegar
Cheese ravioli with marinara sauce

Snack: 1 tangerine

TIP _____

Fresh summer corn on the cob is absolutely delicious just as
nature made it, without butter or salt.

Training Week Three—Sunday

ATTITUDE

1. Smoke ten or fewer cigarettes today, according to
   your plan. Remember, you don't have to cut down
   any further until Quitting-Day. Don't use up too
   many of your ten cigarettes early in the day. The
   hours between 7 P.M. and 11 P.M. are often the most
   difficult. Your index cards will tell you if this is true
   for you.
2. Idle hands get into mischief! You're going to have a
   lot of time on your hands; at least two or three
   hours that you used to spend fiddling with smoking
   paraphernalia are now free. Find something else to
   do with them:
   • Start some needlepoint.
   • Build a model airplane.
   • Knit a scarf.
   • Learn to paint.
   • Plant an herb garden.
   • Teach yourself to play the harmonica.
   • Do a jigsaw puzzle.

- Write a letter.

3. Don't forget to use deep breathing and visualization to get through cravings. As we've said before, if you could see a craving attack, it would look something like a wave, building slowly in intensity, peaking, and then receding. By dealing with each attack as it occurs you are taking control of your habit and avoiding the danger of being caught off-guard.

4. Write in diary: *"Only six days till I'm a non-smoker."*

5. Reward yourself: Call a friend you haven't spoken to for a while; make a date to meet.

EXERCISE
Take the day off.

A day off from exercise once or twice a week allows muscles to recover. Vigorous exercise causes microscopic tears in muscle tissue that take about forty-eight hours to heal.

DIET

Morning
1.
1 cup fresh pineapple chunks
1 bowl oatmeal or other whole-grain hot cereal
1 slice whole-grain toast

Snack: 1 serving yogurt, preferably unsweetened

or

2.
1 whole orange or orange juice

1-egg mushroom omelette
1 piece whole-grain toast

Snack: 1 small bunch grapes

Midday
1.
1 cheese sandwich, broiled, on English muffin or
    whole-wheat bread, with provolone, Swiss, or
    American cheese
Mixed green salad with Vinaigrette*
1 tangerine

Snack: 1 apple, 1 rice cake

or

2.
Tomato stuffed with Crab Salad*
2–4 whole-grain crackers
1 small bunch grapes

Snack: 1 glass apple juice

Evening
1.
3 to 5 ounces broiled salmon
Broiled tomato halves
Broiled whole mushrooms
Romaine-Apple Salad*
½ grapefruit, drizzled with honey and broiled

Snack: Fresh pineapple chunks

or

2.
1 bowl chili con carne
Mixed green salad, Vinaigrette*
French bread or whole-wheat pita bread, brushed
    with olive oil and minced garlic and broiled five
    minutes
1 cup fresh fruit salad
2 oatmeal cookies

Snack: 1 apple

Training Week Three—Monday

ATTITUDE

1. Smoke ten or fewer cigarettes today, according to
   your schedule.
2. Avoid alcohol or try a new drink.
3. Avoid smoky places and smoking people.
4. Don't forget: Always brush your teeth after every
   meal.
5. Keep your hands busy doing something that inter-
   ests you.
6. Write in diary: *"Only five days till I'm a nonsmoker."*
7. Reward yourself: Buy a best-seller.

EXERCISE
Walk twenty minutes.

TIP

Walking is good for thinking and creativity. Aristotle, Plato,
da Vinci, Rousseau, Keats, and Einstein were all avid walkers.

TIP ────────────────────────────

When you start thinking about a vacation, why not plan a fitness holiday? Go someplace with hiking trails, for example. Or go on a canoeing trip or to a dude ranch. Check with your travel agent about the many walking tours that are organized all over the world these days. It will help keep you fit and be a good way to avoid smoking.

────────────────────────────────

DIET

Morning
1.
1 whole orange or orange juice
1 toasted English muffin topped with mashed banana
    and cottage cheese or peanut butter

Snack: 1 apple, 1 glass low-fat milk

or

2.
½ grapefruit or 1 glass grapefruit juice
1 bowl dry cereal with ½ banana
1 piece whole-grain toast

Snack: ½ banana, 3 dried apricots

Midday
1.
1 bowl Crab Bisque*
2–4 whole-grain crackers
Steamed broccoli seasoned with lemon juice and olive
    oil (serve hot or cold), or 8 broccoli flowerets,
    with your choice Low-Fat Dip*
½ papaya

Snack: 2 pieces candied ginger or ⅓ cup raisins

or

2.
1 white-meat turkey sandwich on whole-grain bread
Coleslaw*
1 apple

Snack: any amount carrot sticks and broccoli flowerets, with your choice Low-Fat Dip,* if desired.

TIP _____
A mint "rounds off" the meal and helps curb the urge to smoke.

Evening
1.
Fish Fillets with Garlic-Bread Crumb Topping*
1 baked potato
Red cabbage Coleslaw*
Chocolate Sponge Cake* or 1 bowl fresh cherries

Snack: 2 whole-grain crackers spread with your choice Low-Fat Dip*

or

2.
Sliced roast turkey breast (no more than 2
    tablespoons gravy)
1 cup mashed potatoes or 1 baked sweet potato
1 cup fresh peas
Mixed green salad with Vinaigrette*

Cranberry Upside-Down Cake* or 1 bowl fresh
   pineapple chunks

Snack: 2 pieces candied ginger

Training Week Three—Tuesday

ATTITUDE

1. Smoke ten or fewer cigarettes today, according to
   your plan.
2. Play with worry beads if you start to feel anxious.
3. Use deep-breathing exercises to get through cravings.
4. List in your diary reasons you're glad you smoke
   less and reasons you're nervous about quitting.
6. Write in diary: *"only four days till I'm a nonsmoker."*
7. Reward yourself: Buy flowers for your desk or
   home, or a flower for your buttonhole.

EXERCISE
Walk twenty minutes.

TIP _____
If you work out at dusk or after dark, be sure you wear
reflectors. Front and back reflectors help drivers see you.
Many sports shoes and jackets come with built-in reflective
strips.

TIP _____
Don't push yourself so hard that you remain out of breath for
more than a few seconds after your walk ends. If you are still

trying to catch your breath five minutes after walking, the damage to your heart from years of smoking may be a problem. Check with your physician immediately if this happens to you.

___

DIET

Morning
1.
1 tangerine
1 bowl dry cereal topped with fresh peach or banana
1 slice whole-grain toast

Snack: 1 glass grape juice and a handful of sunflower seeds

or

2.
½ cantaloupe or wedge other melon
1 bowl oatmeal or other hot cereal
1 piece whole-grain toast

Snack: 1 tangerine

TIP ___

Try this unforgettable cure for overeating used by researchers Polivy and Herman to help compulsive overeaters: Crumble up your favorite "temptations" in your hands—cookies, potato chips, chocolate candies, etc.—and drop it all into the toilet. The only difference between flushing it and eating it, say the two researchers, is that when you flush it you bypass the middleman.

Midday
1.
1 small lean beef patty, broiled, with lettuce and
     tomato on whole-grain bread or bun
1 fresh peach or other fresh fruit in season

Snack: 4 leaves romaine lettuce. Tear into pieces as
you go along. Dip each in Low-Fat Dip.*

or

2.
1 cup tomato soup or Cherry Tomato Soup*
2 slices whole-grain bread with 2 thin slices Swiss or
     mozzarella cheese, mustard, lettuce, thinly sliced
     cucumber
Applesauce, preferably unsweetened

Snack: 1 fresh pear or 1 whole orange

Evening
1.
White Bean and Tuna Salad*
1 Artichoke with Yogurt Sauce Verte*
Cherry tomatoes
Poached Peaches in Red Wine and Honey*

Snack: Grapefruit juice

or

2.
3 to 5 ounces broiled halibut or other fish steak
Baked potato topped with yogurt and green onions
Steamed spinach seasoned with lemon
1 Baked Banana*

Snack: 1 rice cake

TIP

Just as visualizing yourself as a nonsmoker helps you to quit, picturing yourself as a slim person encourages you to eat like one.

Training Week Three—Wednesday

ATTITUDE

- Smoke ten or fewer cigarettes today, according to your schedule
- Visualize working without cigarettes. Try a smoke-free afternoon at work today.
- Practice the Clench-Relax exercise from the Fifteen-Minute Survival Kit in Chapter three. Start with the muscles in your face and work down to your toes. This exercise is great whenever you feel anxious or tense.
- Write in diary: *"Only 3 days till I'm a nonsmoker."*
- Reward yourself: Plan a vacation. Pick up travel brochures from a travel agent. There is life after smoking!

EXERCISE

Walk thirty minutes.

TIP

Regular exercise helps keep *you* regular by increasing the muscular contractions of your intestines. There is no such thing as a constipated marathon runner.

TIP

Never take salt tablets or increase your salt consumption, no matter how hot the weather or how hard you think you're working. In order to use up the daily nine to twelve grams of salt most Americans eat, you'd have to produce about three quarts of sweat. Taking extra salt can lead to exhaustion, cramps, and elevated blood pressure.

DIET

Morning
1.
½ grapefruit
1 scrambled egg
½ large or 1 small bran muffin, preferably Blueberry
    Bran Muffins*

Snack: ½ large or 1 small bran muffin

or

2.
½ orange cut in half and eaten with a spoon like a
    grapefruit
1 cup unflavored yogurt with sliced banana
1 rice cracker

Snack: 5 dried apricots, 3 bread sticks

Midday
1.
3 to 5 ounces broiled or poached salmon garnished
    with lemon wedges
Sliced tomato and cucumber
Coleslaw*

whole orange (cut in eighths and peeled)

Snack: a handful of dry cereal (about ⅓ cup)

or

2.
Spaghetti with Fresh Tomato Sauce*
Small salad with lettuce, cucumber, and Vinaigrette*
   oatmeal cookie

Snack: ½ cantaloupe or other melon wedge

TIP _____

Make a double recipe of Fresh Tomato Sauce and store extra
portion in freezer or refrigerator.

Evening

1.
Chicken Breast Scaloppine*
Fusilli or other pasta sprinkled with olive oil and
      parmesan
Mixed green salad
Fresh cherries, or coffee yogurt

Snack: 1 apple

or

2.
Shrimp Salad*
Garnish: lettuce leaves, cherry tomatoes, and your
      choice of other raw vegetables, with your choice
      Low-Fat Dip*

Fresh peach or nectarine, sliced, with frozen vanilla
  yogurt

Snack: 1 glass grape juice or grape juice spritzer (grape
juice with a splash of seltzer)

Training Week Three—Thursday

ATTITUDE

1. Smoke ten or fewer cigarettes today, according to
   your schedule
2. Visualize working successfully without cigarettes.
3. Line up support in advance. If you're giving up with
   someone else, you've already got an ally. If you're
   going it alone, tell your family and friends that what
   you are about to do is difficult. You will need all the
   help you can get.
   Ask them not to:
   • offer you cigarettes.
   • bring ice cream and candies into the house.
   • arrange to meet you in smoky bars or places you
     associate with smoking.
   • tell you they liked you better when you smoked.
   Ask them to:
   • be understanding if you're irritable and short-tem-
     pered.
   • help you with the children so you have time for
     yourself.
   • keep their problems to themselves for a couple of
     weeks.
   • go walking with you.
   • cook meals for you.
   • smoke somewhere else.

4. Plan activities away from places where people are smoking or eating. But don't overdo it. You'll be under a lot of stress, and the less you expect of yourself the easier it will be to deal with it.
5. Write in diary: *"Only two days till I'm a non-smoker."*
6. Reward yourself: Splash on a new perfume or after-shave lotion. Select some good movies from the newspaper or video store to watch this weekend.

EXERCISE
Walk thirty minutes.

TIP _____

Regular exercise can help prevent back pain by strengthening muscles in the pelvis and lower back. It may also protect you from colds. It is common lore among runners that they get fewer colds than their non-running peers. Experts theorize that regular exercise may raise body temperature just enough to provide an inhospitable environment for certain kinds of microbes.

TIP _____

Working up a sweat on your walks? Good—it's a sign that you're getting a workout. Sweating helps to flush nicotine and other toxins from your body.

DIET

Morning
1.
½ grapefruit
1 bowl dry cereal topped with fresh berries or banana
1 slice whole-grain toast

Snack: 1 glass V-8 or tomato juice

or

2.
1 whole orange or orange juice
1 English muffin
2 slices Canadian bacon
Applesauce, preferably unsweetened

Snack: 1 glass low-fat milk

Midday
1.
½ papaya with cottage cheese
½ English muffin or bagel
4 dried prunes

Snack: 1 tangerine, 1 rice cake

or

2.
1 cup split-pea soup
4–5 bread sticks
1 cup mixed fresh fruit salad topped with yogurt

Snack: 5–6 broccoli flowerets, 8 carrot or celery sticks, with your choice Low-Fat Dip.*

Evening
1.
Bluefish with Garlic*
Succotash (corn mixed with lima beans)
Mixed green salad, Vinaigrette*
½ cantaloupe

Snack: popcorn (no oil, no butter)

or

2.
Broiled Chicken Livers with Fresh Tomato Sauce*
Rice, preferably brown rice
Steamed Broccoli with Yogurt Sauce Verte* (use
    artichoke recipe)
2 oatmeal cookies

Snack: apple juice

Training Week Three—Friday

ATTITUDE

1. Smoke ten or fewer cigarettes today, according to
   your schedule.
2. Ignore the voice saying: "Next week is the worst
   week to quit. I've got a big presentation, the kids'
   teeth need fixing, the car is in the shop, and it's
   raining." There's never a "perfect time" to quit.
   Remember, you've made it this far, so onward and
   upward!
3. Review your progress in the past three weeks.
   - You have reduced your nicotine intake substan-
     tially.
   - You have modified your smoking behavior so that
     you now control when and where you smoke.
   - You have improved forever the way you eat and
     take care of your body.
4. HOORAY FOR YOU! You are in very good shape
   to cope with the week ahead. But there is still one

element without which no attempt to change your life can ever be successful: *You must believe that you will succeed!* Dorothy Parker said: "Four be the things I'd been better without: Love, curiosity, freckles, and doubt." It's no good just hoping you'll succeed; you have to be certain. Hope leaves room for doubt. Have confidence in your ability to pull through.

5. Shop this week for next week's food.
   • *Never* go shopping without a written list.
   • *Never* buy anything you haven't decided on in advance.
   • Clear the refrigerator of junk food and sweet things.

6. If you have children in the house, tell them that they will help you by not bringing pizza, candy, ice cream, or other treats into the house. Ask them to be very, very nice to you, even if, for a week or two, you're not particularly nice to them.

7. At the end of the day *throw out everything that reminds you of smoking.* Ashtrays, match books, old packets of cigarettes, and your lighter. Get rid of them all. Break any remaining cigarettes in half. Throw them away. Make a ritual of it; *say good-bye.*

8. Write in diary: *"I have just stubbed out my last cigarette. I am now a nonsmoker. I will not smoke for the next twenty-four hours."*

EXERCISE
Take the day off.

TIP _____
Exercise may be the answer to jet lag. Well-exercised laboratory hamsters subjected to travel-type stress adjusted to new time zones much faster than their sedentary lab-mates. More

and more human travelers are checking into hotel health clubs or tracks as soon as they arrive in a new city.

TIP

Never wear a rubber or plastic "sauna suit" in the hope of losing weight while you exercise. Overheating will just make you tired and may even lead to heat exhaustion.

DIET

Morning
1.
½ cantaloupe
1 cup lemon yogurt
1 toasted bagel

Snack: 1 handful raisins (about ⅓ cup), 1 small handful sunflower seeds

or

2.
½ grapefruit (save other half for snack)
2 small or 1 large bran muffin, preferably Blueberry
    Bran Muffins*

Snack: 1 apple.

Midday
1.
Cold pasta tossed with Vinaigrette* and your choice
    of chopped raw vegetables
1 artichoke with Yogurt Sauce Verte*
1 cup fresh pineapple chunks

Snack: 1 serving yogurt, preferably unsweetened

or

2.
1 Tuna Salad* sandwich on rye or other whole-grain
    bread with lettuce and tomato
Carrot sticks
Coleslaw*
1 cup stewed prunes

Snack: ½ grapefruit

Evening
1.
Gazpacho Soup*
Jalapeño Pepper Pie*
Sliced tomatoes with Vinaigrette*
1 cup fruit salad: sliced kiwis and orange sections

Snack: 1 rice cake

or

2.
1 roasted Cornish game hen
Orzo Baked with Garlic and Cheese*
Mixed green salad, Vinaigrette*
1 tangerine

Snack: 1 glass V-8 juice or tomato juice

Quitting Week—Saturday

ATTITUDE

1. Write in diary: *"I will not smoke for the next twenty-four hours."*
2. Find time to prepare your mind. This week meditate for twenty minutes if you feel your anxiety level starting to rise. Meditation is an excellent way to clear your mind of destructive thoughts and keep you feeling confident and relaxed. Here is a simple meditation exercise to do every day this week.

Meditation Exercise:
- Sit quietly in a comfortable position, with your eyes closed.
- Try and clear your mind as you fix your concentration on the space between your eyes.
- If unwanted thoughts begin to intrude, gently push them away. Don't get upset, just persuade those thoughts to leave. Concentrate on the space between your eyes until your mind is clear.
- Repeat the word "one" to yourself.
- After a few minutes open your eyes. You will feel calm and peaceful. Even two minutes of this meditation can be beneficial. Twenty minutes will set you up for the entire day.

Remember, never force meditation. Like trying to fall asleep, the harder you try, the more difficult it becomes.

3. Use all your new breathing and visualization skills to get through craving attacks.
4. Record in your diary what withdrawal symptoms you are feeling.
5. Reward yourself: Learn a new dance step.

EXERCISE
Walk thirty minutes.

TIP _____

Don't be a fair-weather exerciser. Many beginners use less-than-perfect weather as an excuse to procrastinate and/or give up on exercise. Experienced exercisers learn how to dress properly to protect themselves against cold, rain, or heat. There are, however, exceptions; very high humidity and heat (in the nineties) or very cold weather (temperatures in the teens and below) are appropriate reasons to limit exercise.

DIET
To get you through the quitting week, plan on eating at least two small snacks between each meal as a substitute for cigarettes. You may want to have the morning snacks at 9:30 A.M. and 11:00 A.M. and the afternoon nibbles at 2:30 P.M. and 4:00 P.M. Vary snacks according to your work and meal schedules. Remember, always eat slowly and chew carefully. Make each snack last!

Morning
1.
1 orange (whole or freshly squeezed juice)
1 bowl oatmeal or other hot cereal
1 slice whole-grain toast

Snack 1: grapefruit juice, 3 bread sticks.
Snack 2: small bunch grapes

or

2.
½ cantaloupe
1 egg scrambled with minced chives and parsley

Snack 1: 4 dried apricots, 1 rice cracker
Snack 2: 1 glass apple juice, any amount of raw vegetables of your choice

Midday
1.
1 cup tomato soup or Cherry Tomato Soup*
1 white-meat turkey sandwich on whole-grain bread
    with lettuce
1 tangerine
1 Gingerbread Crisp* or gingersnap

Snack 1: 6 slices raw cucumber or celery
Snack 2: 1 glass low-fat milk

or

2.
Salade Niçoise*
2 bread sticks
1 cup applesauce, preferably unsweetened
1 oatmeal cookie or graham cracker

Snack 1: 1 cup vanilla or unflavored yogurt with sliced
strawberries or banana
Snack 2: "Smoothie"* of your choice

Evening
1.
1 bowl Broccoli Soup*
3 to 5 ounces fresh tuna or other fish steaks, broiled
    or baked

Lima Beans with Garlic*
1 baked apple

Snack 1: small handful raisins (about ⅓ cup)
Snack 2: 3 bread sticks

or

2.
Treat yourself to dinner at your favorite Chinese restaurant.
Chicken or Shrimp with Black Bean Sauce
Broccoli with Garlic Sauce
Rice, preferably brown rice
Fortune cookie

Snack 1: small handful sunflower seeds (about ⅓ cup)
Snack 2: ½ glass low-fat milk.

Quitting Week—Sunday

ATTITUDE
Today is "Why am I doing this?" day. By now you may have forgotten that quitting is something you want to do. You may be thinking of it as something that is being done to you. Someone has forcibly separated you from the cigarettes that you love, the cigarettes that have always made you happy. It isn't fun and it doesn't seem fair.

1. Get out your list of pros and cons. Quitting is worth a few days of discomfort, isn't it?
2. Look on the bright side. *This is total self-indul-*

gence week. During Quitting Week a little self-indulgence isn't just expected, it's required.

3. Have a hot bath; it will relax you and help rid your body of toxins. There is something healing and hedonistic about a long, hot bath. Soak for at least twenty minutes.

4. Distract yourself. Read an absorbing book or knit an absorbing sweater.

5. Give yourself permission to behave badly. Have a tantrum if you want to. Scream! Yell! Pound a pillow! Let out all the anger and frustration you are feeling on the pillow. Really bash it. In minutes you will feel much better.

6. Write in diary: *"I will not smoke for the next twenty-four hours."*

EXERCISE
Walk thirty minutes.

TIP _____

For extra relaxation, distraction, and calorie-burning this week, squeeze in an additional ten to fifteen minutes of walking. Tack it on to your regular program, or find another time during the day to do it. For example, you might try parking your car ten minutes away from work or from the supermarket. Get off the bus a couple of stops early. Instead of going to a restaurant for lunch use the time to go for a walk, stopping for a deli sandwich on the way back to work.

TIP _____

Years of heavy smoking may have damaged your heart without your being aware of it. In addition to shortness of breath persisting for five minutes after exercising, other signs that you may be overtaxing your heart include chest pain, nausea, or dizziness, a pulse rate that remains elevated at 110 beats per minute or higher for fifteen minutes or longer after you stop exercising is also a warning sign. Get in touch with your doctor immediately if you experience any of these symptoms.

***

DIET

Morning

1.
½ cantaloupe
1 large or 2 small bran muffins, preferably Blueberry
    Bran Muffins*

Snack 1: 1 whole orange (peel orange and separate sections)
Snack 2: 2–3 dried prunes, 1 rice cake

or

2.
1 whole orange or orange juice
Fluffy French toast (use 2 slices whole-grain bread in
    1 egg yolk beaten with 2 tablespoons milk, then
    in 1 egg white whipped stiff)

Snack 1: 4 breadsticks, grape juice
Snack 2: 1 wedge raw cabbage, 4–5 strips red or green pepper

Midday

1.
1 can sardines garnished with sliced onion, capers,
    lemon wedges, cherry tomatoes, sliced cucumber
2–4 whole-grain crackers or rice cakes
1 cup fresh pineapple chunks

Snack 1: 1 apple
Snack 2: any amount of raw vegetables of your choice
and Low-Fat Dip.*

or

2.
1 lean beef patty on ½ English muffin or whole-grain
        bun, garnished with mustard, tomato, lettuce,
        sliced raw onion (optional)
Coleslaw*
½ cantaloupe

Snack 1: small bunch grapes, 1 graham cracker or
oatmeal cookie
Sanck 2: 1 tangerine

TIP _____

Instead of ordering dessert, try an espresso or cappucino
instead. That's the pleasant and nonfattening way many Eu-
ropeans round off their meals.

Evening
1.
1 3- to 5-ounce lamb chop, broiled
1 baked potato
Mixed green salad with Vinaigrette*
1 whole peach or pear
2 Gingerbread Crisps* or gingersnaps

Snack 1: popcorn (no butter or oil)
Snack 2: small bunch grapes

or

2.

Spaghetti Putanesca*

Salad with lettuce and an assortment of your favorite
    chopped raw vegetables, Vinaigrette*

1 slice Chocolate Sponge Cake* or 1 cup fresh fruit
    salad

Snack 1: orange juice or orange spritzer (add seltzer to
juice)

Snack 2: small handful dry cereal (about ⅓ cup)

Quitting Week—Monday

ATTITUDE

1. Start the day with twenty minutes of meditation.
2. Visualize a social event without cigarettes, but don't
   lead yourself into temptation yet. Give yourself a
   week before attending a big party or entertaining at
   home.
3. All the little irritations of life that you used to deal
   with by lighting a cigarette may seem unbearable
   this week. Don't let this unexpected anger throw
   you. Use one of your new breathing or visualization
   techniques to relax and let off steam.
4. Ask friends who still smoke to smoke somewhere
   else. They don't mean to be inconsiderate, so don't
   be afraid to ask them nicely not to smoke around
   you. It's possible that the sight of a full ashtray will
   make you crazy this week.
5. Use Milton Feher's deep-breathing technique
   whenever cravings strike.
6. Record all craving attacks and how long they last in
   your diary. How many withdrawal symptoms are

164

you still feeling? How severe are they? Record these, too.

7. Write in diary: *"I will not smoke for the next twenty-four hours."*
8. Reward yourself: Get tickets to a ball game or movie.

EXERCISE
Walk thirty-five minutes.

TIP _____

Do you have an important presentation at work in the near future? Exercise beforehand! By stimulating your circulation and metabolism and elevating your pulse, exercise can make you feel more alert and better able to concentrate.

TIP _____

Review your walking technique periodically. Your arms should swing rhythmically and your legs should move out in long strides. Make a conscious effort to straighten your spine; think of your head as a balloon attached to your spine, floating effortlessly above your neck.

DIET

Morning
1.
½ grapefruit
1 bowl dry cereal with ½ sliced peach or banana
1 slice whole-grain toast

Snack 1: ½ peach or banana, 1 graham cracker
Snack 2: 4 bread sticks, 1 glass water

or

2.
1 whole orange or orange juice
1 bowl oatmeal or other hot cereal
3 dried apricots

Snack 1: 1 whole grapefruit (peel and divide into sections)
Snack 2: ½ toasted bagel, preferably plain, 1 glass low-fat milk

Midday
1.
1 Tuna Melt*
Mixed fresh-fruit salad

Snack 1: 1 serving yogurt, preferably unsweetened
Snack 2: 1 handful sunflower seeds or raisins (about ⅓ cup)

or

2.
1 bowl lentil or mushroom-barley soup
4–5 breadsticks
1 fresh pear, 1 small wedge Brie or Camembert
    cheese

Snack 1: 5 strips raw red or green pepper, 3 broccoli flowerettes
Snack 2: apple juice, 2 Gingerbread Crisps* or gingersnaps

Evening

1.

Broiled Spicy Shrimp and Scallops*
Brown rice or wild rice
Romaine-Apple Salad*
Angel Food Cake* or 1 serving lemon yogurt

Snack 1: whole grain cracker spread with your choice
Low-Fat Dip*
Snack 2: 6 carrot sticks

or

2.

Chicken Breasts with Elephant Garlic*
1 baked sweet potato, topped with spoonful of yogurt
Steamed spinach
Thin slices of fresh orange, drizzled with Grand
     Marnier or other orange liqueur (optional)

Snack 1: 1 serving yogurt, preferably unsweetened
Snack 2: 1 tangerine

Quitting Week—Tuesday

ATTITUDE

1. Start the day with twenty minutes of meditation.
2. Use breathing techniques to get through most cravings. Use the Fifteen-Minute Survival Kit if you can
   take a short exercise break.
3. Don't forget to carry your talisman. Hang onto it in
   meetings and other tense situations.
4. Let out anger and frustration by yelling at the top of

your voice (but don't yell *at* anyone). Let off steam somewhere out of earshot so people don't think you're being murdered.

5. Write in diary: *"I will not smoke for the next twenty-four hours."*

6. Reward yourself: Go dancing or turn up the radio and dance to your favorite song. Dancing is fun, and all that jumping around will make you feel better.

EXERCISE
Walk thirty-five minutes.

TIP

Has giving up cigarettes left you feeling depressed? You may be particularly discouraged now if you don't see visible signs of improved physical fitness after all these weeks of walking. Unfortunately, most of the body changes brought about by exercise—weight loss, toning, muscle tightening, limberness—usually take a couple of months to be noticeable. Don't despair—buy yourself a flattering new pair of walking shorts or a bright-colored T-shirt. Every time you put it on you'll remind yourself that walking is improving your health and helping you kick the smoking habit.

DIET

Morning
1.
½ cantaloupe
1 poached egg
1 slice whole-grain toast

Snack 1: 1 tangerine
Snack 2: 1 handful (about ½ cup) dry cereal

or

2.
1 tangerine
1 bowl dry cereal with ½ banana or fresh strawberries
1 slice whole-grain toast

Snack 1: ½ banana or 3–4 fresh strawberries
Snack 2: 1 rice cake, orange juice

Midday
1.
1 bowl Manhattan clam chowder
2–4 whole-grain crackers or rice cakes
Mixed green salad with Vinaigrette*
Baked apple

Snack 1: 1 glass grape juice
Snack 2: 5 carrot sticks, 4–5 broccoli flowerettes, your
choice Low-Fat Dip*

or

2.
Chicken Salad* garnished with lettuce, tomato, and
    cucumber
1 fresh pear or peach

Snack 1: 3 dried apricots, 1 rice cake
Snack 2: 1 apple

Evening
1.
1 bowl Broccoli Soup,* served cold
3- to 5-ounce chicken breast, broiled

Eggplant Pudding*
Frozen vanilla yogurt (no more than ½ cup, or about
    half of a 5-ounce container)
2 Gingerbread Crisps* or gingersnaps

Snack 1: 6 slices raw cucumber
Snack 2: apple juice

or

2.
Baked Salmon with Capers*
Roast New Potatoes with Garlic and Rosemary*
Steamed green beans
Watermelon wedges or other melon in season

Snack 1: 4 bread sticks
Snack 2: handful sunflower seeds (about ⅓ cup)

TIP _____
Skinless chicken breasts derive 19% of their calories from
fat. Skinless chicken thighs get 47% of their calories from fat.

TIP _____
Lighter dinners keep *you* lighter. Eating heavy meals at the
end of the day when you are inactive lowers metabolism and
leads to weight gain.

Quitting Week—Wednesday

ATTITUDE

1. Start day with twenty minutes of meditation.
2. Visualize a situation where other people are smoking. Make the distinction in your mind between *those* people who are smokers and *you,* a non-smoker. Experience them smoking without wanting to smoke yourself.
3. Write a list of smoking pros and cons. Compare it with your original list.
4. Write in diary: *"I will not smoke for the next twenty-four hours."*
5. Record your feelings and symptoms in your diary. How did you feel today when you saw someone else smoking? Did you resent them or wish you could join them? Did the visualizing exercise change your feelings in any way?
6. Reward yourself: LAUGH! Norman Cousins' *Anatomy of an Illness* turned us all on to the fact that laughter is healing. It makes sense. Laughter is the release of tension. So during this week laugh as much as you can. If nothing strikes you as particularly funny at the moment, rent an old Laurel and Hardy or Charlie Chaplin movie. Buy a joke book.

EXERCISE
Walk thirty-five minutes.

TIP

Need a little humorous inspiration today? Listen to Bill Cosby, who, in spite of reaching middle age, still exercises for

171

both weight control and pleasure. He explains, "I recently turned fifty, which is young for a tree, mid-life for an elephant and ancient for a quarter-miler, whose son now says, 'Dad, I can't run the quarter with you any more unless I bring something to read.'" (*Runner's World*, April, 1988.)

TIP

Guard against sunburned lips and fever blisters. Protect your lips with a lip-care product containing sunblock.

DIET

Morning
1.
½ grapefruit
1 English muffin toasted with thin slice mozarella or
    ricotta cheese

Snack 1: 1 apple
Snack 2: 1 rice cake, handful of raisins

or

2.
½ cantaloupe or other melon
1 large or 2 small bran muffins, preferably Blueberry
    Bran Muffins*

Snack 1: Handful of sunflower seeds
Snack 2: V-8 or tomato juice or grapefruit juice, 4
bread sticks

Midday

1.

Spaghetti seasoned with olive oil, garlic, and
    parmesan
Raw spinach salad with Vinaigrette*
1 cup stewed prunes or figs

Snack 1: ½ cantaloupe
Snack 2: apple juice, handful of sunflower seeds (about
⅓ cup)

or

2.

Grilled Chicken Salad*
1 bowl fresh blueberries or 1 kiwi, sliced

Snack 1: grapefruit juice
Snack 2: your choice "Smoothie"*

Evening

1.

Swordfish with Belgian Endive Sauce*
Steamed spinach sprinkled with 1 tablespoon
    parmesan
Wild rice or brown rice
1 slice Angel Food Cake* with sliced fresh peaches

Snack 1: 4 cherry tomatoes
Snack 2: ½ glass low-fat milk

or

2.
Gazpacho Soup*
Whole-grain crackers with your choice Low-Cal Dip*
1 cup fresh berries with vanilla yogurt
Lemon yogurt

Snack 1: handful of raisins (about ⅓ cup)
Snack 2: 4 bread sticks

Quitting Week—Thursday

ATTITUDE

1. Start the day with twenty minutes of meditation.
2. Review your cards and make a note to avoid people
   and places that you used to associate with smoking.
   As we've said before, much of the urge to smoke is
   association. One look at Ted and all you can think
   of is beer, football, and cigarettes. For a week or two
   stay away from Ted, stay away from football, you
   know the rest.
3. Look at your list of withdrawal symptoms. Cross
   out those you are no longer feeling. Congratulations! You have survived the worst that your addiction could throw at you and lived to tell the tale.
4. Reward yourself: Buy yourself something flattering
   to wear. Something you would hate to grow out of!
5. Write in your diary: *"I will not smoke for the next
   twenty four hours."*

EXERCISE
Walk thirty-five minutes.

TIP _____

Remember to drink plenty of water when you're exercising in warm weather. Don't wait for thirst to take a drink. By that time you may not be able to replace lost fluid.

DIET

Morning
1.
1 orange (whole or freshly squeezed juice)
1 bowl dry cereal with fresh peaches or banana
1 slice whole-grain toast

Snack 1: grapefruit juice, 4 breadsticks
Snack 2: 8 carrot sticks

or

2.
1 poached egg on ½ English muffin
1 bowl mixed fresh fruit

Snack 1: ½ English muffin with ricotta cheese or peanut butter
Snack 2: 1 tangerine

TIP _____

Forgot to bring a snack from home? Find a vending machine that offers fresh fruit or juice. Buy some gum or dried fruit. Avoid nuts. They're usually nutritious, but also very high-calorie.

Midday

1.
3 to 5 ounces of broiled sole or flounder
1 small boiled potato, seasoned with minced parsley
    or dill
Steamed spinach seasoned with lemon juice
Frozen vanilla yogurt (no more than ½ cup)

Snack 1: 1 wedge raw cabbage
Snack 2: 1 rice cake

or

2.
1 white-meat turkey sandwich on whole-grain bread
    with lettuce and sliced tomato
Coleslaw*
1 apple

Snack 1: 5–6 broccoli or cauliflower flowerettes
Snack 2: V-8 or tomato juice

Evening

1.
Chick Pea Cakes with Fresh Tomato Sauce*
Steamed zucchini
Mixed fresh fruit salad

Snack 1: 5–6 broccoli flowerets or 1 cabbage wedge
Snack 2: 1 glass grape juice spritzer (grape juice with a
splash of seltzer)

or

2.
Steamed Mussels in White Wine*
Mixed green salad, oil and vinegar
1 baked apple

Snack 1: 1 glass apple juice
Snack 2: 4 bread sticks

Quitting Week—Friday

ATTITUDE

1. Today you should be feeling more like your old self. CELEBRATE—YOU'VE WON! Plan a party to celebrate your first weeks as a nonsmoker. Schedule it for three weeks from today. Tell all your friends and family so they can congratulate you for quitting.
2. Begin the day with twenty minutes of meditation.
3. Spend more time outdoors. Deep breathing in the fresh air speeds oxygen to your brain.
4. Sing out loud to raise your spirits when cravings strike.
5. Write in your diary: *"I will not smoke for the next twenty-four hours."* Maintain this one-day-at-a-time approach for the next month at least. It will help you avoid overconfidence, which can lead to relapse.

EXERCISE
Take the day off. You've earned it.

TIP
This is a good time to join a walker's club. There are many organizations that sponsor weekly walking clinics, races,

group walks, and other walking events. For information about a walking club in your area check with your local YMCA, runners' club, or the sports editor of your local newspaper.

TIP _____

Planning a get-together with friends or family soon? Suggest a group hike or walk as part of the day's events.

TIP _____

The American Lung Association suggests you learn something new to take the place of smoking. They propose karate or dance classes, for example. Other possibilities include fencing lessons, horseback riding, scuba diving—let your imagination go wild! This is an excellent time to adopt an activity that will keep you fit, bring you pleasure, and give you even more reasons not to smoke.

DIET

Morning
1.
½ cantaloupe
2 slices Canadian bacon
1 scrambled egg
1 slice whole-grain toast

Snack 1: small bunch grapes
Snack 2: V-8 juice or tomato juice or apple juice

or

2.
½ grapefruit
1 bowl yogurt, preferably unsweetened
½ large bran muffin or 1 small, preferably Blueberry
    Bran Muffins*

Snack 1: ½ grapefruit
Snack 2: 6 dried apricots, ½ bran muffin

Midday
1.
Chicken Salad* sandwich on rye bread with lettuce
    and tomato
1 tangerine

Snack 1: 2 Gingerbread Crisps* or gingersnaps
Snack 2: 1 serving yogurt, preferably unsweetened

or

2.
1 cup split-pea soup
1 cup fresh fruit salad with cottage cheese
2–4 whole-grain crackers or rice cakes

Snack 1: 8 carrot sticks
Snack 2: grape juice, handful of raisins (about ⅓ cup)

Evening
1.
Broiled Spicy Shrimp and Scallops*
1 to 2 cups pasta shells tossed with olive oil and
    parmesan cheese
Mixed green salad, oil and vinegar
Cold Coffee Soufflé* or Poached Peaches with Red
    Wine and Honey*

Snack 1: whole-grain cracker spread with ricotta cheese
Snack 2: 1 tangerine

or

2.
Fish Fillets with Garlic-Bread Crumb Topping*
Lima Beans with Garlic*
1 tomato and 1 sliced onion salad tossed with oil and
      vinegar
Choice any amount of raw vegetables of your choice
      with Low-Fat Dip*
Half papaya

Snack 1: 1 rice cake
Snack 2: 1 apple

If you're yearning for an after-dinner cigarette, talk yourself out of it by repeating the little poem written about a hundred years ago by Benjamin Waterhouse:

> *Tobacco is a filthy weed,*
> *That from the devil does proceed,*
> *It drains your purse, it burns your clothes,*
> *And makes a chimney of your nose.*

You've made it! You've successfully carried out your commitment to STOP SMOKING!

7

Maintenance

Attitude Goals

Congratulations. You have survived your first week as a nonsmoker. You probably feel weary, battle-scarred, and tempted to breathe a huge sigh of relief. Don't relax yet.

By now many—indeed, most—of the symptoms of withdrawal will have diminished or disappeared altogether. But old habits die hard, and the time you feel most secure is the time you are most in danger of relapsing.

You have at least three months to go before you have beaten the odds. This is not meant to depress you but merely to keep you vigilant.

ALLOW FOR A PERIOD OF MOURNING

After the initial euphoria of successfully giving up smoking you might be hit with feelings of incredible loneliness. You have, after all, just given up a friend that has probably been with you for most of your adult life. The one that comforted you in times of trouble and congratulated you when you succeeded. It isn't surprising that you feel a little lost without this "friend" around to keep you company. In a very real sense you are in mourning.

These feelings are sometimes the hardest to recognize. Don't let them overwhelm you. Keep busy. Your optimism will return once your brain is convinced it can't fool you into giving it any more lethal drugs. Much of the depression you feel during withdrawal is chemically induced. Your addiction is playing with your emotions to get a "hit" of nicotine.

If you go to a party and suddenly realize you are smoking, you haven't "failed." You've been tripped up by some combination of environmental and social stimuli. You could call it the ex-smoker's Bermuda Triangle, the mysterious force field that sucks back seventy percent of all ex-smokers less than a year after they quit.

DON'T LET A LAPSE TURN INTO A RELAPSE

The minute you light a cigarette after a period of abstinence you start a chain reaction that goes something like this: The nicotine you inhale gives you a greater "lift" because you haven't smoked for a while. This is not an illusion. Your body, no longer adjusted to regular doses of nicotine, reacts with a surge of gratitude that closely resembles your first pleasurable experience with smoking: immediate and powerful relief of anxiety. However, as soon as you are smoking regularly again, your old tolerance level zooms back to where it was before you quit. Cigarettes are once more producing anxiety, not alleviating it. So don't let one slip turn into an excuse to resume smoking.

Remember: one cigarette—*one puff*—and you'll be

re-addicted. Even if you feel *convinced* that you can handle the "special occasion" cigarette, you can't. If that sounds harsh, isn't it better to err on the side of caution? It would be sad to see all your hard work go up in a puff of smoke!

WHO RELAPSES?

According to the U.S. Department of Health and Human Services, you are in danger of relapse if:

• you find dealing with stress very difficult.
• you fail to recognize and deal with the triggers that set off the urge to smoke.
• you have not changed your view of smoking or your view of yourself as someone who is capable of quitting.
• you have inadequate support from your peers.

If you have followed the *Stop Smoking* program diligently, you are in very good shape to deal with all of these relapse traps.

WHAT TRIGGERS RELAPSE?

The farther away you get from the trauma of quitting, the easier it is to become complacent. All the problems you used to cure with cigarettes have not vanished just because you quit smoking. Your best defense is to arm yourself in advance with other methods of coping with your problems. Never be caught off-guard. Here is a list of relapse "triggers":

You've Had a Fight with Your Mate

He or she has been mean and rotten, and you want to have a cigarette just out of spite. Walk around the block. Punch a pillow. Take ten deep breaths. Talk about the problem. By tomorrow you'll have kissed and made up. But if you light up, you'll just have to quit smoking all over again.

You're at a Party Drinking and a Cigarette Jumps into Your Hand

Don't panic. Calmly stub it out and make a point to be especially vigilant in social situations.

As you know, alcohol weakens your resolve. Don't test yourself until you feel ready. Be on your guard at all times.

You Live with Someone Who Smokes

Flush with success, you may experience the common phenomenon of ex-smoker's backlash. This does not take the form you would expect. Instead of feeling sorry for your former fellow smokers, you resent them. Suddenly, you can't stand the sight of a dirty ashtray or the smell of smoke on your loved one's clothes.

As a nonsmoker you feel superior to the "poor fools" who are still enslaved. You've beaten it; why can't they? Remember what pride comes before? Don't risk a fall. Throughout the entire ordeal of quitting smoking there are little mine fields of overconfidence. You *think* you've got it licked. You *think* one puff of a friend's cigarette won't hurt you. This kind of thinking is especially dangerous if your smoking friend lives with you because all day you smell smoke and see smoking paraphernalia.

Your newfound hostility is only a thin disguise for desperate longing. Beg your friend to smoke somewhere else. Designate a nonsmoking room in your home where you'll be safe.

There Are Smokers at the Table

After a meal, watching them light up and smelling the smoke can be a powerful incentive to smoke yourself. Excuse yourself when you have finished eating. Brush your teeth. Do not return until they have stopped smoking.

Stress

An article in *The Journal of Consulting and Clinical Psychology* in December 1985 cites stress as the most important reason for failure to quit smoking. The article also says that successful abstainers "use more self-reward strategies and positive self-statements than less successful subjects."

So continue to reward yourself and write yourself encouraging notes in your diary. If you feel shaky, recommit yourself by writing: *"I will not smoke for the next twenty-four hours."* Do this every day, if necessary.

One of the first things to do when you feel things are getting a bit out of control is to talk the problem over with a friend. Don't be afraid to tell your troubles to someone else. Let them know you'll be more than happy to listen to their woes in return. Didn't Grandma ever tell you that a problem shared is a problem halved?

You Feel Bored, Anxious, and Depressed

People get bored and depressed when they feel helpless. The way to cure depression is not to suck it down with a cigarette, but to take positive action to change the situation that is depressing you. *The opposite of anxiety is not tranquility; it is the perceived ability to control your life.*

187

Smoking only gave you the *illusion* of control. In reality, as a smoker you were totally dependent on and controlled by cigarettes. You exchanged self-control for immediate relief from anxiety. Without cigarettes you really are in control. Now all you need to do is effectively manage anxiety. You don't have to get rid of it altogether; a little lets you know you're alive. Just manage it.

The *Stop Smoking* program has given you several specific ways to manage stress: relaxation, deep breathing, meditation, exercise, and diet. All of these techniques will help you *enjoy* life as a nonsmoker.

Exercise Goals

More and more health professionals and fitness experts are recommending walking as the best form of exercise for people of all ages. As we said before, ordinary nonstop, brisk walking is an efficient, injury-free way to maintain fitness, improve cardiovascular health, and control weight. If you keep up the walking program you embarked on when you gave up cigarettes, you'll not only feel better and look better than you did before, but you'll be less apt to want to smoke. A healthy body is more pleasurable than one that's addicted to nicotine. To maintain a healthy level of cardiovascular fitness and muscle strength it is necessary to walk a minimum of thirty minutes a day, at least three days a week.

OTHER FORMS OF WALKING
If you are in fairly good shape and eager for a vigorous workout that burns more calories than ordinary walking, you might try one of the more athletic forms of walking.

Health-Walking or Fitness-Walking

Health-walking is just vigorous walking with an exaggerated arm swing. Set a swift pace, swing your arms purposefully, and stride forward with shoulders down and head high. Maintain a brisk, steady pace for at least thirty minutes.

Racewalking

This Olympic sport is becoming increasingly popular with people of all ages. This "funny" arm-swinging way of walking is fun and unlike jogging or regular walking, has the advantage of building upper-body as well as lower-body strength. Your local library has books about racewalking, and many communities offer free instruction clinics. With these simple instructions you can try it out on your own:

Step forward on the heel of your left foot, keeping your left leg straight. Pull your right leg forward, keeping it straight, and place it down heel first. Keep your arms loosely bent and close to your sides. Pump your arms vigorously as you move forward. Think of your legs as poles pulling you along. This all feels awkward at first, but with practice a comfortable rhythm sets in. Remember, the leg moving forward is straight-kneed. Don't deliberately swing your hips from side to side the way some racewalkers appear to do; this is a movement that occurs naturally as you begin to get the hang of it and start moving forward more rapidly.

"By moving your arms like a sprinter, you can move faster, which will raise your heart rate higher than normal walking," explains Howard Jacobson, president of the Walkers Club of America. Racewalking lets you use more muscles and burn more calories than jogging, with less risk of injury.

TRIATHLON ACTIVITY

The triathlon approach—engaging in several different sports rather than sticking to a single activity—has become popular with fitness experts. Originally promoted as an endurance marathon where competitors raced in an arduous program of bicycling, running, and swimming, the idea of mixing activities is now being adopted by people of all levels of fitness, age, and skill. You can put this strategy to good use by mixing your activities in any number of different ways:

1. Add another exercise to your existing program—say, walking in the morning and playing tennis later in the day, after work. Or join a health club and ride the exercycle for twenty minutes, swim twenty minutes, and work out on the machines for another twenty minutes. Increasing the length of time you work out helps you avoid weight gain.
2. Alternate activities each day. Perhaps you want to stick with a walking program but find it tedious to go out day after day doing the same old thing. If you're feeling fit now, take up raquetball or squash. Join a YMCA or health club with a pool. Sign up for a dance class. Then figure out a workable schedule. For example, you might walk thirty minutes to work on Monday and Wednesday mornings, play ball on Tuesday and Thursday evenings, and go to a dance class on Friday. You might add a game of golf (no cart!) or tennis on the weekend. The important thing is to decide on a schedule and stick to it. Many people find that paying for a health club membership or for athletic lessons is a strong economic incentive to keep active.

The triathlon approach has distinct advantages:

Variety

Varying your exercise program is a good way to prevent boredom. Keeping your interest up helps you stick with it.

Work More Muscles

A variety of activities exercise more muscles than the pursuit of a single sport. Jogging, for example, mainly works certain leg and ankle muscles, doing virtually nothing for your upper body. But if you also swim a couple of days a week, chest and arm muscles will become strong and well-shaped, too. Or alternate an aerobic dance class (preferably low-impact) with a walking program to burn calories and give most of your muscles an efficient workout.

Fewer Injuries

Single-sport activities place constant wear and tear on the same muscles day after day. Varying your exercise allows specific muscle groups the opportunity to recover. Remember, before you start any new exercise program, consult your physician.

AEROBIC EXERCISE

Aerobic exercise is the process of maintaining a level of activity long enough and with enough intensity for oxygen to be converted to energy. Here's how it works. When the oxygen you inhale is combined with stored food substances called glycogen, energy is produced. The stored food is burned off in the process.

If the period of activity is too brief or two slow for the oxygen to be used this way, the exercise is called anaerobic, meaning "without oxygen." Exercise that consists of stops and starts—for example, bowling, calisthenics, golf, and tennis—is usually anaerobic exercise. Jogging, brisk continuous walking, bicycling, and other activities that allow the heart rate to accelerate and *stay* at the increased rate for an extended period of time are aerobic exercises.

Both aerobic and anaerobic forms of exercise are valuable. Both should be practiced for maximum fitness. Both have the capacity to burn calories.

Anaerobic exercise is particularly good for strengthening muscles and for developing coordination and limberness. Aerobic exercise not only works muscles but also strengthens the cardiovascular system. Aerobic exercise provides other benefits as well by:

- lowering blood lipids, which remove fat from the blood and push it into the muscle, where it is used for energy.
- increasing the oxygen-carrying capacity of the bloodstream.
- enabling the body to burn more calories (and, according to recent studies, continue to burn calories at an accelerated rate for several hours after exercise has ended).

When Is It Safe to Begin Aerobic Exercise?

The vessel walls of your heart are beginning to repair themselves now that you've quit smoking, but the process can be very slow. Unfortunately, there is no way to determine just how much damage may have been done to your heart when you smoked. If you were a light smoker, are in good health, and are under the age of forty, it is probably safe to begin more vigorous aerobic exercise within the first few months after quitting. Before you begin an aerobic program, check with your doctor.

Ex-smokers over forty who are not in excellent

health, or who were heavy smokers, should not undertake an aerobic exercise program without first consulting their physicians. It may be at least a year, and as many as five years, before your heart recovers enough to safely withstand vigorous aerobic work.

How to Reach an Aerobic Level

The common-sense way to know if you're getting the cardiovascular benefits of your workout depends on how you feel. If you push yourself a little, work up a sweat, and maintain a fairly steady level of activity for at least thirty minutes, you're getting a good workout.

If you'd like to know exactly how hard you're working, a standard formula for judging aerobic levels has been developed.

- Subtract your age from 220. This is your maximum heart rate.
- Determine what sixty to seventy-five percent of that rate should be. This is your exercise *target zone*.
- Take your pulse about five minutes after beginning exercise. To do this, place your index and third fingers over the inside of your wrist or elbow, or against the large vein at the side of your neck (press very gently here so that you don't impede circulation in the carotid arteries). Count the beats for one minute.

For example, if you are forty years old, subtracting your age from 220 gives you a maximum heart rate of 180. Sixty to seventy-five percent of 180 is 108–135 beats per minute. That is what your pulse should be after five minutes of an aerobic workout. If your pulse is faster, you are pushing your heart rate out of the safe zone—*slow down*. If your pulse falls below the target zone, you push a little harder to achieve aerobic benefits.

CAUTION: EXERCISE CAN BE OVERDONE

A word of warning: Some ex-smokers channel their former smoking compulsion into exercise fanaticism. As more people take up exercise to lose weight, a compulsive addiction to *thinness* has become prevalent. Professional coaches report that lately they've seen anorexic men as well as women working out. "Toothpicks with a great set of lungs" is the way Bob Sevene, advisor to the Nike Boston team, described people who use exercise to keep their weight below normal. Don't jump on the national weight-obsession bandwagon. Set realistic weight goals for yourself, then use exercise to maintain them.

Diet Goals

The *Stop Smoking* program demonstrates that diet and exercise can work in tandem to keep your metabolic rate high enough to avoid the weight gain brought on by smoking cessation. By continuing to follow the dietary principles set forth in the training period—a low-fat, low-sugar, high-fiber and high-complex carbohydrate diet—chances are good that you won't gain weight now that you've passed the most critical period of quitting smoking.

What if you *have* gained weight over the past four weeks? If you're concerned that you've put on a little weight in spite of following the exercise and diet programs, you may now have to take a closer look at your eating habits. But first, take a careful look at your weight to make sure you really have put on unwanted pounds.

TRACKING YOUR WEIGHT

Refer back to the records you kept of your weight during the first week of the training period. Next weigh yourself, remembering to do so at the same time of day, dressed in the same way. If your weight is within three to five pounds of what it was then, don't worry. Remember that the average healthy person's weight varies by a few pounds from day to day, depending on such factors as hormonal fluctuation and fluid retention.

If you find yourself weighing five or more pounds over your average weight of that first week, you may wish to correct the situation right now. The way to do that is to examine what brought on the weight gain in the first place.

WHAT SHOULD I WEIGH?

Expert opinion varies on ideal weights for healthy adults. The Metropolitan Life Insurance Company offers an index most health professionals accept, but others feel it errs on the heavy side. Still others worry that the index doesn't take into consideration individual variances and the fact that muscle weighs more than fat, so fit people with considerable muscle mass may legitimately weigh more than less-active people.

Scales are not really an accurate measurement of healthful weight. Almost everyone agrees that measuring body fat is more important than measuring how much you weigh. There are formulas for pinching your skin in order to measure inches of fat behind the arm or on the abdomen. But these aren't really reliable guides either. A device called the skinfold caliper is used by many nutritionists and sports trainers to measure the amount of fat under the skin. Some fitness experts recommend that you measure your waist, upper arms, and hips and keep track of fluctuations in these mea-

METROPOLITAN HEIGHT AND WEIGHT TABLES

All weights are in pounds for adults 25 to 59 years old. Men's weights and heights include clothing weighing 5 pounds and shoes with 1-inch heels. Women's weights and heights include clothing weighing 3 pounds and shoes with 1-inch heels.

MEN

Height	Small Frame	Medium Frame	Large Frame
5-2	128-134	131-141	138-150
5-3	130-136	133-143	140-153
5-4	132-138	135-145	142-156
5-5	134-140	137-148	144-160
5-6	136-142	139-151	146-164
5-7	138-145	142-154	149-168
5-8	140-148	145-157	152-172
5-9	142-151	148-160	155-176
5-10	144-154	151-163	158-180
5-11	146-157	154-166	161-184
6-0	149-160	157-170	164-188
6-1	152-164	160-174	168-192
6-2	155-168	164-178	172-197
6-3	158-172	167-182	176-202
6-4	162-176	171-187	181-207

WOMEN

Height	Small Frame	Medium Frame	Large Frame
4-10	102-111	109-121	118-131
4-11	103-113	111-123	120-134
5-0	104-115	113-126	122-137
5-1	106-118	115-129	125-140
5-2	108-121	118-132	128-143
5-3	111-124	121-135	131-147
5-4	114-127	124-138	134-151
5-5	117-130	127-141	137-155
5-6	120-133	130-144	140-159
5-7	123-136	133-147	143-163
5-8	126-139	136-150	146-167
5-9	129-142	139-153	149-170
5-10	132-145	142-156	152-173
5-11	135-148	145-159	155-176
6-0	138-151	148-162	158-179

Source: 1979 Build Study, Society of Actuaries and Association of Life Insurance Medical Directors of America, 1980, © 1983 Metropolitan Life Insurance Company

MEASURING YOUR FRAME SIZE WITH YOUR ELBOW

To determine your frame size, bend the forearm upward at a 90-degree angle. Keep the fingers straight and turn the inside of your wrist toward the body. Place the thumb and index finger of your other hand on the two prominent bones on either side of your elbow. Elbow measurements below are for men and women of medium frame. Measurements lower than those listed indicate you have a small frame while higher measurements indicate a large frame.

MEN

Height (in 1-inch heels)	Elbow breadth (inches)
5'2"–5'3"	2½"–2⅞"
5'4"–5'7"	2⅝"–2⅞"
5'8"–5'11"	2¾"–3"
6'0"–6'3"	2¾"–3⅛"
6'4"–	2⅞"–3¼"

WOMEN

Height (in 1-inch heels)	Elbow breadth (inches)
4'10"–4'11"	2¼"–2½"
5'0"–5'3"	2¼"–2½"
5'4"–5'7"	2⅜"–2⅝"
5'8"–5'11"	2⅜"–2⅝"
6'0"–	2½"–2¾"

Source of basic data: National Health and Nutrition Survey, 1971–75, National Center for Health Statistics, © 1983 Metropolitan Life.

surements in order to monitor healthy weight and body size.

For a rough idea of average weights and heights, consult the Metropolitan Index. For a more accurate assessment of where your weight should be, consult your physician.

The Overactive Sweet Tooth

Studies show that many ex-smokers have an increased craving for sweets. If you suspect this has happened to you, don't eat dessert for the next ten days. Rely on fresh fruit to satisfy your desire for something sweet. Yearning for a candy bar? Try a glass of apple juice or a handful of blueberries instead. You may be surprised at how much the natural sugar in fruits can satisfy that desire for something sweet. If your weight begins dropping by the end of ten days, you'll know that you must be vigilant about your sugar intake in the future.

Bolster your confidence with the reminder that craving sweets is linked to craving cigarettes, and that the urge for both will pass with time. By the end of three months it will have subsided. After the first year your increased craving for sugar will have normalized as long as you've been careful not to substitute a sugar habit for a nicotine habit.

CHARTING YOUR EATING PATTERNS

Persistent weight gain even when desserts have been reduced may be caused by the most common problem of all, eating too much. Many ex-smokers aren't even aware that they overindulge. The best way to stick to reasonable eating patterns is to use the behavioral techniques that worked to get you off cigarettes. Just as you altered certain thought patterns and changed your habits in order to quit smoking, you can also change the ways you think about food and diet.

Encouraging a positive approach to changing the way people think about smoking and eating is favored by Herbert Spiegel, a psychiatrist and teacher at Columbia University's College of Physicians and Surgeons. The negative way of looking at a habit you're trying to break—saying "Don't do this, don't do that"—leads easily to failure, according to Dr. Spiegel.

"For example, if I say to you, 'Don't think about purple elephants,' what's the first thing your mind conjures up? Purple elephants, of course. In the same way, as soon as someone tells you, 'Don't smoke,' suddenly smoking is the only thing you can think about," Dr. Spiegel told us in an interview.

Instead of concentrating on the reasons you shouldn't smoke, Dr. Spiegel uses hypnosis to help patients tap into the positive side of their desire to give up smoking. The same positive frame of mind, he says, can be used in thinking about the way you eat. Learn to think in terms of protecting your body and taking care of it with a good diet. With practice, following a nutritious diet becomes less something you *should* do, and more what you *want* to do. You'll want to eat right and stay trim and healthy.

AVOIDING RELAPSE

"I kissed my first woman and smoked my first cigarette on the same day," Arturo Toscanini claimed. "I have never had time for tobacco since."

For most people, forgetting about cigarettes takes a little longer than it did for Toscanini—anywhere from three months to a year. These critical three to twelve months are full of traps. Sometimes relapse occurs when stress builds up to the point where you feel you just can't get through another day without smoking. At other times relapse comes out of the blue. One night at a party after a couple of drinks, there you are, dancing on top of the piano with a lampshade on your head and a cigarette in your hand.

Do these lapses mean you've failed? No. The goal of the attitude, exercise, and diet techniques you learned during the *Stop Smoking* program will help you to deal with situations such as these. As we've explained before, one of the major causes of relapse is weight gain. "Cigarette companies have taken advantage of this for years," the American Lung Association explains in a pamphlet called "Stop Smoking/Stay Slim." "They want you to smoke as a way of controlling weight and coping with life's pressures. Regardless of the consequences." Armed with the advice from the *Stop Smoking* program, you won't be fooled.

The tendency to gain weight may persist from three weeks to up to a year after quitting smoking. A 1986 University of California at San Francisco study shows that weight gain may continue up to the twenty-sixth or fifty-second week after quitting, depending on how heavy a smoker you were. With healthy exercise and diet you can sidestep this trap. Exercise and healthy eating will help you control weight and develop the attitudes and habits of fit nonsmokers. Feeling trim, fit, and healthy is a deterrent to smoking. And improved health is one of the great benefits of giving up cigarettes. You'll soon feel that way yourself.

8

Smoking and Pregnancy

"Cigarette smoking and pregnancy simply are not compatible," according to New York obstetrician Richard Hausknecht. Approximately a third of women of childbearing age are smokers. Studies show that about a third will quit, a third will cut down, and a third will continue to smoke as usual during pregnancy. According to *Cancer: Facts and Figures,* a booklet published in 1988 by the American Cancer Society, a Federal Trade Commission staff reporter found that fifty percent of women do not know that smoking during pregnancy increases the risk of stillbirth and miscarriage. In fact, there is almost nothing more hazardous to your pregnancy than smoking.

The emotional upheavals experienced during and after pregnancy—weepiness, moodiness, depression—may be felt more keenly without cigarettes to rely on. On the other hand, maternal instinct is such a powerful drive that mothers-to-be may be motivated enough to quit smoking with relatively little effort. If you're pregnant and you feel your resolve to give up cigarettes begin to weaken, just think about the dire consequences of smoking for your baby's health. Your determination to quit, at least during pregnancy, may be stronger than ever.

Two constituents of cigarette smoke pose an immediate threat to the fetus: carbon monoxide and nicotine. By binding to the hemoglobin in the pregnant woman's red blood cells, carbon monoxide hinders the exchange of oxygen and carbon dioxide between mother and fetus. Nicotine causes, among other things, spasm of blood vessels, resulting in reduced blood flow to the pregnant uterus. What are the possible consequences? Low birth weight, which is the major cause of death for newborns. Premature placenta separation is also a hazard. There is new evidence linking some behavioral difficulties and intellectual deficiencies in children to smoking during pregnancy.

WHEN TO QUIT

The safest bet, in terms of family planning, is to give up cigarettes before conception. The first trimester is the most critical in terms of fetal development. And if you wait until you're pregnant to quit, both you and the baby will have to go through the trauma of withdrawal.

If you didn't know you were pregnant, or if you haven't been able to quit before, the earlier you stop during the pregnancy the better, as far as your baby's health is concerned. If you're pregnant, the time to quit is now.

If you've smoked all through your pregnancy, you can at least reduce the risk of oxygen deprivation during childbirth by not smoking again until after delivery.

NURSING MOTHERS

Would you willingly force a spoonful of milk contaminated by nicotine and other dangerous toxins into your newborn infant's mouth? Breastfeeding mothers who smoke are doing just that. Toxic substances from cigarettes pass through the mother's bloodstream directly into her milk. Babies and young children are particularly susceptible to the poisons they inhale in the form of "passive smoke" from their mothers' cigarettes. If you haven't stopped smoking yet, improve your baby's chance for a healthier life by quitting now.

EXERCISE

Discuss exercise with your obstetrician. A regular exercise program is usually recommended for pregnant women. Not only will exercise help keep you in shape, but it may also contribute to keeping your metabolism and hormonal levels on as even a keel as possible during pregnancy. By helping you to stay limber, exercise may make delivery easier. Working out will also distract you from the urge to smoke. Nursing mothers will get back into shape much sooner if they exercise regularly.

The bouncy, jerky movements of conventional aerobics classes are usually contraindicated for pregnant women, but low-impact activities such as walking or swimming are considered safe. Swimming is probably the ultimate exercise for a pregnant woman because it is a non–weight bearing activity. There are also many special exercise classes for expectant mothers offered by health clubs, the YMCA, or other community activity centers.

If you are setting up your own program, take it slowly and don't ever push beyond a pace you can easily manage. Try to be consistent—it's a *regular* exercise program, not a strenuous one, that will help compensate for the metabolic disturbances a pregnant woman may experience when she gives up smoking.

DIET

Fear of gaining weight is definitely not a valid excuse for the pregnant woman to continue smoking. You would have to gain over fifty pounds before it could be considered a hazard equal to smoking for both mother and child. Gaining too little weight during pregnancy is usually a greater problem than too much. If you are pregnant, it is twice as important to follow a nutritionally sound, low-fat diet; you are eating for two. After checking it out first with your obstetrician, you can use the menus and recipes in this book, or follow your own practitioner's guidelines for a diet high in complex carbohydrates and low in fat and sugar. Most obstetricians recommend a diet composed of approximately forty to fifty percent complex carbohydrates, twenty-five percent protein, and no more than twenty percent fat.

Drink plenty of water to help flush out toxins and avoid constipation.

ALCOHOL

Like nicotine, alcohol is a drug. The best time for mothers-to-be to give up alcoholic beverages is before conception. Heavy drinkers (five to six glasses of beer, wine, or liquor per day) have up to a fifty percent greater risk of having a baby with symptoms ranging from mental retardation, skeletal malformations, central nervous system disorders, to abnormalities of the heart, urogenital tract, or facial structure.

Although the evidence isn't entirely clear, even moderate drinking seems to complicate pregnancy.

Since no one really knows the effects of drinking on fetal development, most experts recommend that a pregnant woman give up all alcohol. Think of it this way: Every drink you have goes through your bloodstream, through the placenta, and into your developing baby. While our own livers have a capacity for detoxifying the results of moderate alcohol consumption, the fetus's does not. The results for your baby can be severe.

If you are pregnant and haven't given up alcohol before now, remember: The chances of having a healthy baby decrease the longer you continue drinking. If you find yourself unable to give up drinking while you're pregnant, consult your obstetrician and ask for recommendations of organizations that may help you.

9

Recipes

ANGEL FOOD CAKE

Angel food cake must be what they had in mind when they came up with the notion of eating your cake and having it too. Since angel food cake is mostly air, with no egg yolk or butter, it's a light 125 calories or so per serving.

    1 cup flour
    1¼ cups sugar
    1½ cups egg whites (about 1 dozen eggs)
    2 teaspoons cream of tartar
    1½ teaspoons vanilla

1. Preheat oven to 375°.
2. Stir together flour and ½ cup sugar.
3. In a separate bowl, beat egg whites until fluffy.
4. Beat in cream of tartar, then add remaining sugar gradually, beating until stiff peaks form.
5. Fold in vanilla.
6. Fold in flour/sugar mixture ½ cup at a time.
7. Pour into an ungreased tube pan with removable bottom.
8. Bake at 375 for 30–35 minutes.
9. Invert pan on funnel or bottle to cool.

ARTICHOKES WITH YOGURT SAUCE VERTE

4–6 medium artichokes

Sauce:
½ cup mayonnaise
½ cup unflavored yogurt
6 scallions (green onions)
½ tablespoon minced parsley
1 tablespoon lemon juice
⅛ teaspoon cayenne pepper
1 tablespoon capers (optional)

1. At least 3 hours before serving trim stems and snip off sharp points of artichokes.

2. Steam artichokes or simmer, covered, in 4–5 inches of water, about 40 minutes, until tender. Test for doneness by pulling out a leaf. If it comes out fairly easily and the fleshy part is tender to the bite, the artichokes are done.

3. Drain thoroughly and chill.

4. Mix together all remaining ingredients (may be done up to 24 hours in advance.

5. Refrigerate at least 2 hours before serving so that flavors can meld. Serve bowl of sauce separately. Serves 4.

BAKED BANANAS

Per person:
1 whole banana
1 teaspoon honey
dash cinnamon

1. Preheat oven to 350°.
2. Peel banana and place in a square of foil measuring about 8 × 6 inches.
3. Drizzle banana with honey and sprinkle with cinnamon. Seal foil around banana.
4. Bake for 20–30 minutes, or until bananas are soft but still hold their shape.
5. Serve warm.

BAKED SALMON WITH CAPERS

Per person:
1 salmon steak or fillet (¼–½ pound)
½ teaspoon soy sauce
¼ teaspoon dill
1 teaspoon capers

1. Preheat oven to 400°.
2. Arrange salmon in a baking dish lined with foil. Rub soy sauce over the top and sprinkle with dill. Sprinkle capers over the top.
3. Bake, uncovered, at 400° for 20 minutes, depending on thickness of salmon. When done, fish should be lightly browned on top and opaque-pink in center.

BLUEBERRY BRAN MUFFINS

This is a hearty, healthy, easy-to-make recipe. The muffins keep well in the refrigerator, or you can make a double recipe and freeze some. We've used raspberries as well as blueberries.

1 cup whole-wheat flour
1 cup bran
1 teaspoon baking soda
½ teaspoon cinammon
¼ cup melted butter
½ cup unflavored yogurt
⅓ cup honey
1 egg
1 ripe banana, mashed
1 cup fresh or frozen blueberries
⅓ cup raisins (1½-ounce box) (optional)
2 tablespoons chopped walnuts or sunflower seeds (optional)

1. Preheat oven to 350°.
2. Stir together flour, bran, baking soda, and cinammon.
3. In a separate bowl, stir together butter, yogurt, honey, and the egg.
4. Combine liquid and dry ingredients, stirring until blended, but being careful not to overmix.
5. Stir in mashed banana and fold in berries, raisins, and nuts as desired. Divide among lightly buttered (or nonstick) muffin pans and bake for 45 minutes. Makes 12 small muffins.

BLUEFISH WITH GARLIC

2 pounds bluefish fillets (or fresh tuna, mackerel,
    salmon or other dark, flavorful fish)
2 large cloves garlic
2 teaspoons lemon juice
2 teaspoons soy sauce

1. Preheat oven to 350°.
2. Arrange fish on a baking sheet lined with foil.
3. Combine remaining ingredients and spoon over fish.
4. Bake for 10 minutes, or until fish is opaque throughout. Serves 4.

BROCCOLI SOUP

This is a simple-to-make, nutritious, low-calorie soup that is equally good hot or cold.

1 medium bunch broccoli
1 medium onion
4 cups chicken broth or water
¼ teaspoon curry powder
½ cup yogurt

1. Chop broccoli and onion coarsely.
2. Place in a large pot along with chicken broth and simmer, uncovered, until broccoli is tender, about 8–10 minutes.
3. Stir in curry powder.
4. When cool enough to handle, transfer ingredients to blender or food processor, in batches small enough to fit. Purée until smooth.
5. Stir in yogurt. Reheat carefully if necessary, or chill several hours or overnight and serve the soup cold. Serves 4.

BROILED SPICY SHRIMP AND SCALLOPS

½ pound unpeeled shrimp
½ pound scallops
1 tablespoon Worcestershire sauce
3–4 cloves garlic, minced
1 teaspoon lemon juice
1 tablespoon red pepper flakes

1. Preheat broiler.
2. Rinse shrimp quickly under cold water but do not peel. Prick each of them two or three times with a fork. If using sea scallops, cut them in quarters.
3. Combine remaining ingredients in a shallow bowl and stir in shellfish. Let marinate, stirring occasionally, at least 1 hour and up to 8 hours.
4. Spread shellfish in a single layer in a broiling pan lined with foil. Broil about 10 minutes, turning once, or until scallops are just opaque throughout. Serves 2.

CHERRY TOMATO SOUP

2 1-pint baskets of cherry tomatoes
1 medium onion, chopped
2 cups chicken broth
1 cup water
1 teaspoon thyme
½ teaspoon basil

1. Rinse tomatoes and remove stems.
2. Place tomatoes in a pot along with remaining ingredients.
3. Simmer 10–15 minutes, or until onions are soft.
4. Transfer mixture to a food processor and purée. Serve hot or cold. Garnish with a spoonful of yogurt or a sprinkling of parsley. Serves 4.

CHICK PEA CAKES WITH FRESH TOMATO SAUCE

About 2 cups cooked garbanzo beans or 2 10½-ounce
    cans chick peas
3 cloves garlic, chopped
2 tablespoons chopped parsley
1 teaspoon chili powder
¼ teaspoon red pepper flakes

1. Preheat oven to 375°.
2. Place all ingredients in blender or food processor and purée until smooth.
3. Divide mixture into quarters and form into four patties or cakes.
4. Arrange on a foil-lined baking sheet and bake at 375° for about 15 minutes, or until lightly browned.
5. Serve with Fresh Tomato Sauce* spooned around cakes. Serves 2 to 4.

CHICKEN BREASTS WITH ELEPHANT GARLIC

Elephant garlic is that oversized garlic—5 to 6 times the size of regular garlic cloves—that is showing up in markets more frequently these days. It is much milder than the usual garlic, with a pleasant, bitterish flavor and buttery texture. You can make this recipe with 3 or 4 cloves regular garlic, but the flavor won't be quite the same. This recipe, by the way, is another extraordinarily simple but satisfying dish.

For each person:
½ boneless, skinless chicken breast
2 cloves elephant garlic

1. Place each piece of chicken in the center of a piece of aluminum foil.
2. Peel garlic, cut each clove in half, and place over chicken.
3. Close foil up over chicken and bake in a hot (425°) oven for about 15 minutes.
4. Open up the foil and finish cooking until chicken and garlic brown a little, about 5–8 more minutes.

CHICKEN BREASTS WITH FRESH CORIANDER SAUCE

Fresh coriander is one of those herbs about which few people feel indifferent—you either love it or hate it. Don't try to use dried coriander, which has an entirely different taste.

Serve the chicken with its vibrant green sauce over brown rice or pasta. Steamed or raw carrots or sliced tomatoes would be a good and colorful accompaniment.

1 whole boneless, skinless chicken breast
1 cup water
¼ cup fresh coriander leaves
1 large clove garlic, chopped
1 tablespoon olive oil
grated parmesan cheese

1. Place chicken breast in a skillet with 1 cup water. Cover and simmer until done, or about 15–20 minutes.

2. Remove chicken to a platter.

3. Turn heat up under skillet and cook broth, uncovered, over high heat for a minute or two, or until mixture is reduced to approximately 1 cup.

4. In a blender or food processor, place coriander leaves, garlic, and olive oil. Process until coriander and garlic are finely minced.

5. Add mixture to chicken broth.

6. To serve, cut chicken breast in half and place each half on a bed of rice or pasta. Pour sauce over chicken. Top with cheese. Serves 2.

CHICKEN BREASTS MARINATED WITH OREGANO

2 skinless, boneless chicken breasts (1½–2 pounds total)
1 tablespoon olive oil
1 tablespoon lemon juice
2 cloves garlic, finely minced
1 teaspoon oregano
½ teaspoon dried pepper flakes

1. Cut chicken in 1-inch cubes. Reserve.
2. Combine remaining ingredients. Toss chicken in marinade, cover, and refrigerate several hours or overnight.
3. Pre-heat broiler.
4. Place chicken in a single layer in a shallow baking dish or pie pan.
5. Broil, turning occasionally, for 7–10 minutes or until chicken is lightly browned and cooked clear through. Serves 4.

CHICKEN BREAST SCALOPPINE

Per person:
½ boneless chicken breast, fat and skin removed
1 teaspoon flour
2 teaspoons olive oil
2 scallions (green onions), sliced
2 large mushrooms, sliced
¼ cup chicken stock
2 tablespoons marsala

1. Sprinkle chicken on both sides with flour and pound with a kitchen mallet or edge of a sturdy saucer until it is very thin (about ¼ inch).
2. Using just enough oil to coat the bottom of a heavy skillet, lightly brown the chicken on both sides.
3. Add scallions and mushrooms and cook over low heat, shaking pan occasionally, for about 1 minute.
4. Pour in chicken stock, cover pan, and simmer until chicken is done, about 10 minutes.
5. Remove chicken to a plate and keep warm.
6. Add marsala to stock, turn up heat, and cook until reduced by about half. Pour over chicken.
7. Sprinkle with parsley, if desired, and serve immediately.

CHICKEN OR SEAFOOD SALAD

Cooked chicken, turkey, tuna, salmon, and fresh or canned shrimp or crab all make delicious and non-fattening salad and sandwich mixtures. There are any number of different optional ingredients, including chopped celery, minced scallions, a dash of curry powder, or a teaspoonful of capers. Adding a little yogurt to the mayonnaise helps reduce the fat and calorie content.

Filling for 1 sandwich:
⅓ cup coarsely chopped cooked chicken
1 tablespoon mayonnaise
1 tablespoon unflavored yogurt

Combine all ingredients.

CHICKEN WITH CHILIES

6–8 whole large dried chilies (such as "California Chili
Pods," available in many markets selling regional
foods)
1 fryer or roasting chicken (3½ to 4 pounds)
½ teaspoon whole black peppercorns
4 whole cloves
3–4 cloves garlic
½ teaspoon cumin
¼ cup red wine vinegar

1. Pull as much fat and skin off chicken as possible and discard.

2. Place dried chilies in a bowl and add enough warm water to cover. Let sit at least 10 minutes.

3. Place chilies, peppercorns, cloves, garlic, cumin, and vinegar in blender or food processor and purée until as smooth as possible.

4. With a table knife, spread mixture all over chicken. Let sit at least 1 hour; overnight would be even better.

5. Bake chicken at 350° for 1½ hours, or until juices run clear when chicken is pricked. If chili coating begins to burn, cover chicken loosely with foil. Serves 6.

CHOCOLATE SPONGE CAKE

Since sponge cakes contain virtually no fat they tend to be lighter in calories as well as texture. This one, which serves 8 people, has about 150 calories per serving—not bad for cake. If you've never made a cake from scratch, try it. You'll be surprised to find that it's just about as easy as opening a box and preparing a mix.

¾ cup unbleached flour
⅓ cup unsweetened cocoa powder
3 eggs
½ cup granulated sugar
½ teaspoon vanilla
3 tablespoons water
2 tablespoons powdered sugar (optional)

1. Preheat oven to 375°.
2. Butter a 9-inch cake pan and line the bottom with a lightly buttered round of waxed paper.
3. Stir together flour and cocoa.
4. In a separate bowl beat the eggs until light and lemon-colored. Gradually beat in the granulated sugar and continue beating until pale and creamy. Beat in vanilla and water.
5. Carefully fold half the flour mixture in, then the other half.
6. Pour the batter into the pan, spreading it evenly all around.
7. Bake for 25–30 minutes.
8. Let cool for 5 minutes, then turn out on a rack.
9. Sift powdered sugar over top if desired.

COLD COFFEE SOUFFLÉ

This is a cool and festive way to end a meal when the weather's warm. Fresh raspberries or strawberries go well with it.

1 cup very strong coffee (may be made with 2 table-spoons instant coffee plus 1 cup boiling water)
1 packet unflavored gelatin
1 tablespoon cold water
¼ cup boiling water
1¼ cups instant nonfat milk powder
6 tablespoons sugar
1 teaspoon vanilla
3 tablespoons rum or brandy (optional)

1. Refrigerate coffee (or place in freezer) until thoroughly chilled.
2. Stir gelatin into 1 tablespoon cold water.
3. Add ¼ cup boiling water and stir until dissolved. Let cool to room temperature.
4. Place chilled coffee in a bowl and sprinkle in powdered milk. Beat until thick. Gradually beat in sugar. Scrape down sides of bowl.
5. Beat in vanilla, gelatin, and rum. Scrape down bowl and beat mixture another minute.
6. Pour into a lightly oiled mold and refrigerate several hours or overnight. Serves about 10.

COLESLAW

There are dozens—no, hundreds—of different ways to make coleslaw. Green or red cabbage may be used. Choose vinaigrette or a mayonnaise-based dressing. Season with dill, caraway seeds, mustard seeds, or a sprinkling of paprika. Grated carrot, minced onion, chopped apple, and sunflower seeds are all popular additions. Coleslaw may be made in advance and kept refrigerated for up to two days. Since cabbage is high in vitamins and low in calories, why not enjoy coleslaw on a regular basis? Here's a very simple recipe to get you started.

> 1 small head green cabbage
> ⅓ cup mayonnaise
> ⅓ cup unflavored yogurt
> 1 tablespoon lemon juice
> 1 teaspoon dried dill

1. Cut cabbage in quarters, trim out hard core, and rinse sections.
2. Shred cabbage with a large knife or with shredding attachment of food processor. Transfer to a large bowl.
3. In a small bowl, whisk together mayonnaise, yogurt, lemon juice, and dill. Pour over cabbage and mix throughly. If mixture seems dry, add another tablespoon each of mayonnaise and yogurt and a few more drops lemon juice.

CRAB BISQUE

   2 medium potatoes, peeled and quartered
   1 medium onion, minced
   1 clove garlic, minced
   2 cups water
   ½ cup white wine
   2 tablespoons tomato paste
   ½ teaspoon basil
   ½ teaspoon paprika
   1 pinch saffron
   dash of cayenne
   8 ounces crabmeat
   2 tablespoons dry sherry (optional)

1. Place potatoes, onion, garlic, and water in a saucepan. Simmer, covered, for 15 minutes, or until potatoes are soft.

2. Add all remaining ingredients except sherry. Simmer, uncovered, for 10 minutes.

3. Carefully transfer mixture to blender or food processor and puree.

4. Return to saucepan, add sherry, and reheat over very low heat just before serving. Serves 4.

CRANBERRY UPSIDE-DOWN CAKE

As cakes go, this variation on a traditional upside-down skillet cake has relatively modest amounts of butter, sugar, and eggs. It's a cinch to make, and an attractive and tasty treat to serve around holiday time.

¼ cup butter
1⅓ cups unbleached flour
2 teaspoons baking powder
¾ cup sugar
1 egg
½ teaspoon vanilla extract
½ cup milk

Topping:
¼ cup butter
1 cup light brown sugar
2 cups fresh or frozen cranberries

1. Preheat oven to 350°.
2. Cream together butter, flour, baking powder, and sugar.
3. Beat in egg, vanilla, and milk. Continue beating until very smooth.
4. Melt ¼ cup butter in a 10-inch iron skillet.
5. Stir in brown sugar.
6. Remove from heat and distribute mixture evenly over bottom of skillet.
7. Spread cranberries over the top.
8. Pour in batter and bake 25–30 minutes.

EGGPLANT PUDDING

1 large eggplant
2 cloves garlic, chopped
1 tablespoon lemon juice
2 shakes Tabasco
2 eggs
½ cup milk
1 large tomato
2 tablespoons parmesan

1. Cut the unpeeled eggplant in slices about 2 inches thick.

2. In enough water to just cover, steam or simmer until tender, or about 8 minutes.

3. Place garlic, lemon juice, Tabasco, eggs, and milk in blender or food processor.

4. Add cooked eggplant and blend thoroughly.

5. Pour into a lightly buttered baking dish or soufflé mold. Slice tomatoes and arrange over top. Sprinkle with cheese.

6. Bake, uncovered, until browned and bubbly, or about 40 minutes. Serves 4 as a main course, 6 as a vegetable dish.

FISH FILLETS WITH GARLIC-BREADCRUMB TOPPING

This light, aromatic breadcrumb topping is a far cry from the heavy breaded and fried fish of fast food chains. It is very low in fat, a snap to make, and best served with something grainy, like brown rice or kasha, and steamed broccoli or a green salad.

1½ pounds flounder or other mild fish fillets
1 slice whole-wheat bread
1 clove garlic, minced
1 teaspoon olive oil
2 tablespoons fresh parsley leaves
4 lemon wedges

1. Arrange the fish in a single layer on a baking sheet.
2. Place all remaining ingredients except lemon wedges in blender or food processor and pulverize. Sprinkle over fish.
3. About 20 minutes before serving, preheat broiler.
4. Broil fish about 10–15 minutes, depending on thickness of fillets. Fish is done when opaque. Serves 4.

FRESH TOMATO SAUCE

1 tablespoon olive or other vegetable oil
1 medium onion, minced
2 cloves garlic, minced
2 medium tomatoes, chopped
1 small (6-ounce) can tomato juice
1 teaspoon basil
¼ teaspoon thyme

1. Place oil in a heavy skillet and warm it over medium heat.
2. Add onions and cook a couple of minutes.
3. Stir in garlic. Cook for 5 minutes, then add tomatoes.
4. Stir in tomato juice and herbs and simmer for 10 minutes, or until tomatoes are very soft and mixture is beginning to soften a little.

GAZPACHO SOUP

1 cup tomato juice
½ cucumber, peeled and coarsely chopped
½ bell pepper, coarsely chopped
1 scallion, sliced
1 whole tomato, coarsely chopped
2 cloves garlic, minced
2 tablespoons wine vinegar
dash cayenne

Place all ingredients in blender or food processor and purée until vegetables are minced. Serve cold. May be made up to 24 hours in advance. Serves 2–4.

GINGERBREAD CRISPS

These melt-in-the-mouth cookies have a delicate flavor that will satisfy your urge for sweets. Keep them in the freezer and eat only one or two at a time.

½ cup butter
½ cup sugar
½ cup honey or molasses
1 egg
1 teaspoon baking soda
1 tablespoon milk
1 teaspoon powdered ginger
1 teaspoon cinnamon
2¾ to 3 cups unbleached flour

1. Cream together butter and sugar.
2. Beat in molasses or honey and the egg.
3. Dissolve baking soda in milk and stir into mixture.
4. Stir ginger and cinnamon into flour.
5. Beat flour mixture into the batter.
6. Chill dough overnight.
7. On a floured surface, roll chilled dough out as thinly as possible.
8. Cut with cookie cutter (or an upside-down juice glass) and arrange on baking sheets.
9. Bake in a preheated 350° oven for 6–8 minutes, or until firm but not too brown.
10. Remove from baking sheets immediately. Makes 4 dozen cookies.

GRILLED CHICKEN SALAD

1 boneless chicken breast, skin and fat removed
3 cups shredded salad greens (choose at least two:
    romaine, arugula, raddichio, endive, watercress)
2 tomatoes, quartered
2 tablespoons blue cheese (optional)
6–8 Mediterranean-style black olives (optional)
1 recipe Vinaigrette*

1. Cut chicken breast in 8–10 strips. Broil or sauté the strips (in nonstock pan, no oil) until cooked through, 5–8 minutes.

2. Arrange salad greens on a serving plate. Top with warm chicken strips and tomato slices.

3. Crumble blue cheese over the top of the salad and add olives, if desired.

4. Spoon Vinaigrette over each portion. Serve immediately. Serves 2.

JALAPEÑO PEPPER PIE

2 canned jalapeño chilies
4 eggs
⅔ cup milk
3¾ ounces farmer or ricotta cheese
2 tablespoons coarsely chopped cheddar or Jack cheese
2 teaspoons chili powder
½ to 1 teaspoon red pepper flakes

1. Preheat oven to 350°.
2. Rinse the chilies under cold water and mince them.
3. Beat the eggs.
4. Combine all ingredients and pour into an oiled 9-inch pie pan.
5. Bake at 350° for 40 minutes, or until pie is firm in center. Serves 4–6.

LIMA BEANS WITH GARLIC

> 2 10-ounce packages lima beans
> 1 tablespoon olive oil
> 2–3 cloves garlic, minced
> 2 teaspoons grated parmesan cheese

1. If possible, defrost lima beans slightly before using (keep them in the refrigerator overnight or leave them at room temperature for an hour or two). Otherwise, put them in the skillet in a frozen block over very low heat, watching carefully and separating them with a fork to make sure they don't burn.

2. Place oil in a skillet (preferably heavy, such as cast iron) and warm it over low heat about 30 seconds.

3. Stir in lima beans and cook, uncovered, over very low heat for 10 minutes, stirring occasionally.

4. Add garlic and continue cooking, stirring occasionally, until tender and lightly browned, for 15 more minutes. If limas become very dry, add another teaspoon oil.

5. Before serving, reheat lima beans and stir in parmesan. Serves 4 to 6.

LOW-FAT DIPS

HUMMUS

> 1 cup cooked chick peas or garbanzo beans (cook according to package direction, or use canned)
> 1 tablespoon olive oil
> 2 tablespoons lemon juice
> 1–3 cloves garlic, minced
> dash cayenne

1. If using canned beans, pour into a colander and rinse in cold water first.
2. Combine all ingredients in blender or food processor and purée until smooth.
3. If a thinner mixture is desired, beat in a tablespoon or two of cold water.

MUSTARD-YOGURT DIP

> 1 cup unflavored yogurt
> 2 teaspoons Dijon-type mustard
> ¼ teaspoon dried dill

Place all ingredients in a bowl and stir until thoroughly mixed.

WHITE BEAN DIP

> 1 cup cooked beans (cook according to package directions, or use canned)
> ¼ cup unflavored yogurt
> 1 tablespoon lemon juice
> 2 tablespoons chopped parsley

1. If using canned beans, place in a colander and rinse under cold water.
2. Combine all ingredients in blender or food processor and purée until smooth.

NEW POTATOES ROASTED WITH GARLIC AND ROSEMARY

If the skins are very thick and tough, peel the potatoes. But they'll have more flavor, more vitamins, and provide more fiber if you leave the skins on.

1 pound small red or yellow potatoes (about golf-ball size)
1 clove garlic, finely minced
1 tablespoon olive oil
1 teaspoon rosemary

1. Preheat oven to 400°.
2. Scrub potatoes, leaving skins on, then steam or simmer them until tender.
3. Transfer potatoes to a bowl and toss gently with remaining ingredients.
4. About 20 minutes before serving, arrange potatoes on a baking sheet.
5. Bake in a 400° oven about 20 minutes, or until very hot and beginning to brown lightly. Serves 4.

ORZO BAKED WITH GARLIC AND CHEESE

3–4 cloves garlic
2 tablespoons olive oil
2 tablespoons lemon juice
1 cup chicken broth
4 cups cooked orzo
½ cup grated parmesan

1. Preheat oven to 350°.
2. In a large skillet, cook garlic in oil over low heat for 2 minutes, or just long enough for garlic to soften but not brown.
3. Remove skillet from heat and stir in lemon juice and chicken broth.
4. Stir in cooked orzo.
5. Transfer half the mixture to a 6–8 cup baking dish. Sprinkle with half the cheese, add the remaining orzo, and top with remaining cheese.
6. Bake, covered, at 350° for 45–50 minutes, or until very hot and just beginning to brown around the edges. Serves 4 to 6.

POACHED PEACHES IN RED WINE AND HONEY

> 4 ripe peaches
> 1 cup red wine
> 1 tablespoon honey
> 2 tablespoons thinly sliced almonds

1. Peel peaches, cut in halves and pit. Slice into ½-inch pieces.
2. Place wine and honey in a skillet and bring to boil.
3. Add peaches and simmer, covered, for 4 minutes.
4. Remove peaches with a slotted spoon and reserve.
5. Turn heat up under wine mixture and boil, uncovered, until mixture is reduced by half, or about 2–3 minutes.
6. Allow to cool slightly, then pour over peaches.
7. Refrigerate until thoroughly chilled, at least 2 hours.
8. To serve, arrange peach slices in a fan shape on each of 4 dessert plates. Spoon wine sauce over them.
9. If desired, spread almonds in a shallow pan and toast them in broiler until brown; scatter them over peaches. Serve as is, or add 2 tablespoons plain yogurt or puréed fresh or frozen raspberries (strained if you don't want the seeds) to each plate. Serves 4 to 6.

ROMAINE-APPLE SALAD

1 small head romaine lettuce
1 whole red or green apple
2 tablespoons olive oil
1 tablespoon unflavored yogurt
1 tablespoon wine vinegar
1 clove garlic, finely minced
1 teaspoon Dijon-type mustard
Freshly ground black pepper

1. Rinse lettuce and pat dry. Tear into bite-sized pieces and place in a salad bowl.
2. Cut unpeeled apple into 1-inch pieces and place in bowl.
3. Combine remaining ingredients and pour over salad, tossing well. Serves 4 to 6.

SALADE NIÇOISE

This is a modified and very simple version of Provence's special salad. We've left out the traditional boiled potatoes and hard-boiled eggs, but if you have any leftover cooked potatoes, by all means slice them into the salad. A few raw peas, sliced radishes, or cooked asparagus spears would also add flavor.

> 1 small head leaf lettuce (Boston, Bibb, or butter, for example)
> 1 7-ounce can water-packed or other white-meat tuna
> 2 medium tomatoes, cut in quarters
> 1 cucumber, sliced (peel if desired)
> 6–8 black olives, preferably Mediterranean-type (optional)
> 1 recipe Vinaigrette*

1. Rinse lettuce leaves and pat dry. Arrange them in a single layer on serving plate or in a shallow bowl.

2. Break up tuna with a fork and scatter over lettuce. Garnish with tomato quarters, cucumber slices, and black olives.

3. Just before serving, pour vinaigrette over salad. Serves 2.

SMOOTHIES

These satisfying and nutritious drinks are easy to whip up in a blender or food processor. Use the following recipes as a guideline, then put your imagination to work and experiment with other ingredients. Fruit juices or low-fat milk make a good base; then add fresh berries, peaches, pineapple, or other seasonal fruits. Cut fruit in chunks for easy blending. Add more liquid for a thinner drink.

SMOOTHIE I
    ½ cup low-fat milk
    3–4 fresh strawberries (or ½ banana)
    ½ teaspoon vanilla
    1 teaspoon wheat germ (optional)

SMOOTHIE II
    ½ cup apple juice
    ½ banana
    1 tablespoon instant powdered milk (optional)

SMOOTHIE III
    ½ cup orange juice
    ½ banana (or 1 fresh peach)

SMOOTHIE IV
    ½ cup milk
    2 tablespoons unflavored yogurt
    ½ banana (or 3–4 fresh berries or other fresh fruit)

SPAGHETTI PUTANESCA

Roughly translated as "Whore's Spaghetti," this Italian favorite is derived from the specialty Neapolitan hookers dished up. This version is quite simple, and you don't even have to cook it. Try it with the new imported sun-dried tomatoes that come in a tube, like toothpaste—it's wonderful! Regular tomato paste works fine, too. Although this dish is low in fat, capers and olives are salty, so if you're on a severely sodium-restricted diet—well, leave them out. You'll still have a wonderful, spicy tomato sauce. The sauce may be made several hours or up to one day in advance.

2 tablespoons tomato paste
3–4 cloves garlic, minced
4 tablespoons olive oil
4 tablespoons hot water
6 ounces tomato juice
½ teaspoon red pepper flakes (or more, to taste)
2 tablespoons capers
¼ pound olives, preferably Mediterranean-type, pitted
   and halved
4 tablespoons pasta-cooking water
1½ pounds spaghetti or other pasta
Parmesan cheese

1. In a bowl, stir together all ingredients except the pasta cooking water, the pasta, and the parmesan.
2. Just before serving, cook the pasta according to package directions. Before draining it, stir 4 tablespoons of the boiling water into the sauce.
3. Drain pasta, transfer it to a serving bowl, and pour sauce over it. Serve parmesan separately. Serves 4 to 6.

STEAMED MUSSELS IN WHITE WINE

2 quarts fresh mussels
2 cloves minced garlic
½ cup white wine
juice of ½ lemon
¼ cup minced parsley

1. Wash mussels and scrape off "beards," if necessary.

2. Combine remaining ingredients in the bottom of a deep pot. Add mussels.

3. Cover and simmer a few minutes (depending on size of mussels) until the shells open.

4. Transfer mussels to individual serving bowls, spooning some of the cooking broth over each. Serves 4–6.

SWORDFISH WITH BELGIAN ENDIVE SAUCE

4 swordfish or halibut steaks (2 to 2 ½ pounds)

The sauce:
2 heads Belgian endive
2 cloves garlic, minced
2 teaspoons vegetable oil
1 teaspoon lemon juice
½ cup milk
½ cup white wine

1. Preheat broiler.
2. Arrange fish on a foil-lined broiling pan or shallow baking dish.
3. To make the sauce, trim and slice endive and cook, along with garlic, in vegetable oil over low heat.
4. When endive is beginning to soften, stir in lemon juice and cook another minute.
5. Add milk and wine and simmer for 10 minutes, or until endive is very soft (mixture will probably curdle slightly).
6. Transfer mixture to a food processor or blender and purée.
7. Meanwhile, broil or grill fish until done.
8. Divide fish among 4 serving plates and drizzle sauce around each piece of fish. Serves 4.

TUNA OR CRAB MELT

1 small can or ⅓ cup white-meat tuna or crabmeat,
   preferably water-packed
1 English muffin (2 halves)
¼ teaspoon dill (optional)
2 thin slices mozzarella, Swiss, or other cheese

1. Drain liquid from canned seafood.
2. Arrange English muffin halves on a baking sheet and divide tuna between them.
3. Sprinkle with dill and top with cheese.
4. Toast in broiler or toaster oven 5–7 minutes, or until cheese has melted.

For variety:
• Add sliced tomato.
• Instead of tuna or crab, use 3–4 stalks cooked asparagus on each muffin half.
• Use rye bread instead of English muffins.
• Experiment with seasonings—try paprika or minced fresh herbs.

VINAIGRETTE

3 tablespoons oil, preferably olive
1 tablespoon wine vinegar
salt and pepper to taste

Whisk all ingredients together and pour over salad.

For variety:
- add 1 clove finely minced garlic
- whisk in 1 teaspoon whole-grain or Dijon-type mustard
- substitute 1 tablespoon tomato juice for one of the tablespoons of oil
- substitute 1 tablespoon yogurt for one of the tablespoons of oil
- add 1 tablespoon chopped fresh parsley or other fresh herbs

WHITE BEAN AND TUNA SALAD

Vinaigrette:
¼ cup olive oil
2 tablespoons wine vinegar
1 clove garlic, minced
½ teaspoon basil

1½ cups cooked white beans (or 1 can cannellini beans, drained)
1 7-ounce can white-meat tuna packed in water
1 red onion, minced
freshly ground black pepper
2 tablespoons minced fresh parsley
fresh basil leaves (optional)

1. Pat beans dry with a paper towel. Make sure beans are well drained.
2. To make the vinaigrette, whisk together oil, vinegar, garlic, and basil.
3. Pour half the mixture over the beans. Toss gently and let marinate at least one hour, if possible.
4. Just before serving, top the beans with the flaked tuna and cover with remaining vinaigrette.
5. Garnish with onions, parsley, and fresh basil leaves. Serves 2.

Suggested Reading

Bennett, William I., and Stephen E. Goldfinger, eds. *Your Good Health: How To Stay Well, and What to Do When You're Not*. Cambridge: Harvard University Press, 1987.

Bennett, William I., and Joel Gurin. *Dieter's Dilemma*. New York: Basic Books, 1982.

Benyo, Richard, and Rhonda Prevost. *Feeling Fit in Your Forties*. New York: Atheneum, 1987.

Brody, Jane. *Jane Brody's Nutrition Book*. New York: W. W. Norton & Co., 1981.

Connery, Donald, with Herbert Spiegel. *The Inner Source: Exploring Hypnosis*. New York: Holt, Rinehart and Winston, 1986.

Cooley, Denton A., and Carolyn E. Moore. *Eat Smart for a Healthy Heart Cookbook*. Woodbury, NY: Barron's, 1987.

Cooper, Kenneth H. *Running Without Fear*. New York: Bantam, 1986.

Desowitz, Robert S. *The Thorn in the Starfish: The Immune System and How It Works*. New York: W. W. Norton, 1967.

Eisenberg, Arlene, Heidi Markoff, and Sandee Hathaway. *What to Eat When You're Expecting*. New York: Workman Publishing, 1986.

Ferguson, Tom. *The Smoker's Book of Health*. New York: Putnam, 1987.

Suggested Reading

Fonda, Jane. *Jane Fonda's New Workout & Weight Loss Program*. New York: Simon & Schuster, 1986.

Gawain, Shakti. *Creative Visualization*. New York: Bantam, 1978.

Goor, Ron, and Nancy Goor. *Eater's Choice: A Food Lover's Guide to Lower Cholesterol*. Boston: Houghton Mifflin, 1987.

Harington, Geri. *Real Food/Fake Food and Everything in Between*. New York: Macmillan, 1987.

Jacobsen, Michael F. *The Fast Food Guide: What's Good, What's Bad, and How to Tell the Difference*. New York: Workman Publishing, 1986.

Milkman, Harvey, and Stanley Sunderwirth. *Craving for Ecstasy: Consciousness and Chemistry of Escape*. Lexington, MA: D.C. Heath and Co., 1987.

Miller, William R. *The Addictive Behaviours: Treatment of Alcoholism, Drug Abuse, Smoking and Obesity*. Elmsford, NY: Pergamon, 1980.

Nagler, Willibald, and Irene von Estorff. *Dr. Nagler's Body Maintenance and Repair Book*. New York: Simon & Schuster, 1987.

Ogle, Jane. *The Stop Smoking Diet*. New York: M. Evans, 1981.

Polivy, Janet, and Peter C. Herman. *Breaking the Diet Habit*. New York: Basic Books Inc., 1983.

Pritikin, Nathan, with Patrick McGrady, Jr. *The Pritikin Program for Diet and Exercise*. New York: Bantam Books, 1980.

Restak, Richard. *The Brain*. New York: Bantam Books, 1984.

Solomon, Neil. *Stop Smoking, Lose Weight*. New York: Putnam, 1981.

Spodink, Jean Perry, and Barbara Gibbons. *The 35-Plus Diet for Women*. New York: Harper & Row, 1987.

The Encyclopedia of Psychoactive Drugs. New York: Chelsea House Publishers, 1985.

The Joy of Quitting: How to Help Young People Stop Smoking. New York: Collier, 1979.

Underwood, Greer. *The Enlightened Gourmet*. Chester, CT: Globe Pequot Press, 1986.

Walford, Roy L. *The 120-Year Diet: How to Double Your Vital Years.* New York: Simon & Schuster, 1987.

Weiss, Herman. *Quit Smoking in Thirty Days.* New York: Bantam, 1984.

Williams, Marcia Sabate. *The No Salt, No Sugar, No Fat, No Apologies (Pritikin) Cookbook.* Trumansburg, NY: Crossing Press, 1986.

Yanker, Gary D. *The Complete Book of Exercisewalking.* New York: Contemporary Books, 1983.

Quitting Smoker's Diary

Quitting Smoker's Diary

_____

_____

_____

_____

_____

_____

_____

_____

_____

_____

_____

_____

_____

_____

_____

_____

_____

_____

_____

_____

_____

_____

Quitting Smoker's Diary

_____
_____
_____
_____
_____
_____
_____
_____
_____
_____
_____
_____
_____
_____
_____
_____
_____
_____
_____
_____
_____
_____
_____

Quitting Smoker's Diary

Quitting Smoker's Diary

_____
_____
_____
_____
_____
_____
_____
_____
_____
_____
_____
_____
_____
_____
_____
_____
_____
_____
_____
_____
_____

Quitting Smoker's Diary

_____
_____
_____
_____
_____
_____
_____
_____
_____
_____
_____
_____
_____
_____
_____
_____
_____
_____
_____
_____
_____
_____
_____

Quitting Smoker's Diary

Quitting Smoker's Diary

_____

_____

_____

_____

_____

_____

_____

_____

_____

_____

_____

_____

_____

_____

_____

_____

_____

_____

_____

_____

_____

_____

Quitting Smoker's Diary

_____
_____
_____
_____
_____
_____
_____
_____
_____
_____
_____
_____
_____
_____
_____
_____
_____
_____
_____
_____
_____
_____